2013
YEAR BOOK OF
**PLASTIC AND
AESTHETIC SURGERY**™

The 2013 Year Book Series

Year Book of Anesthesiology and Pain Management™: Drs Chestnut, Abram, Black, Gravlee, Lien, Mathru, and Roizen

Year Book of Cardiology®: Drs Gersh, Cheitlin, Elliott, Gold, Graham, and Thourani

Year Book of Critical Care Medicine®: Drs Dries, Zanotti-Cavazzoni, Latenser, Martinez, Rincon, and Zwank

Year Book of Dermatology and Dermatologic Surgery™: Dr Del Rosso

Year Book of Diagnostic Radiology®: Drs Elster, Abbara, Oestreich, Offiah, Rosado de Christenson, Stephens, and Strickland

Year Book of Emergency Medicine®: Drs Hamilton, Bruno, Handly, Minczak, Mullin, Quintana, and Ramoska

Year Book of Endocrinology®: Drs Schott, Apovian, Clarke, Eugster, Meikle, Oetgen, Ovalle, Schteingart, and Toth

Year Book of Hand and Upper Limb Surgery®: Drs Yao, Adams, Isaacs, Lee, and Rizzo

Year Book of Medicine®: Drs Barker, Garrick, Gersh, Khardori, LeRoith, Panush, Talley, and Thigpen

Year Book of Neonatal and Perinatal Medicine®: Drs Fanaroff, Benitz, Donn, Neu, Papile, and Van Marter

Year Book of Neurology and Neurosurgery®: Drs Klimo, Minagar, Gandhi, House, Kevill, Liu, Mazia, Panagariya, Ragel, Riesenburger, Robottom, Schwendimann, Shafazand, Uhm, and Yang

Year Book of Obstetrics, Gynecology, and Women's Health®: Drs Dungan and Shulman

Year Book of Oncology®: Drs Arceci, Bauer, Chiorean, Gordon, Lawton, Murphy, Thigpen, and Tsao

Year Book of Ophthalmology®: Drs Rapuano, Cohen, Flanders, Hammersmith, Milman, Myers, Nagra, Nelson, Penne, Pyfer, Sergott, Shields, Talekar, and Vander

Year Book of Orthopedics®: Drs Morrey, Huddleston, Rose, Swiontkowski, and Trigg

Year Book of Otolaryngology-Head and Neck Surgery®: Drs Sindwani, Balough, Franco, Gapany, and Mitchell

Year Book of Pathology and Laboratory Medicine®: Drs Raab and Bissell

Year Book of Pediatrics®: Dr Stockman

Year Book of Plastic and Aesthetic Surgery™: Drs Miller, Boehmler, Gosman, Gutowski, Ruberg, Salisbury, and Smith

Year Book of Psychiatry and Applied Mental Health®: Drs Talbott, Ballenger, Buckley, Frances, Krupnick, and Mack

Year Book of Pulmonary Disease®: Drs Barker, Jones, Maurer, Spradley, Tanoue, and Willsie

Year Book of Sports Medicine®: Drs Shephard, Cantu, Feldman, Galea, Jankowski, Janssen, Lebrun, and Nieman

Year Book of Surgery®: Drs Copeland, Behrns, Daly, Eberlein, Fahey, Huber, Klodell, Mozingo, and Pruett

Year Book of Urology®: Drs Andriole and Coplen

Year Book of Vascular Surgery®: Drs Moneta, Gillespie, Starnes, and Watkins

2013

The Year Book of PLASTIC AND AESTHETIC SURGERY™

Editor-in-Chief

Stephen H. Miller, MD, MPH

Clinical Professor of Surgery and Family Medicine (non-salaried), University of California San Diego, San Diego, California

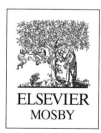

ELSEVIER
MOSBY

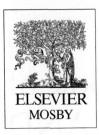

ELSEVIER
MOSBY

Vice President, Continuity: Kimberly Murphy
Editor: Joanne C. Husovski
Production Manager, Electronic Year Books: Donna M. Skelton
Electronic Article Manager: Mike Sheets
Illustrations and Permissions Coordinator: Dawn Vohsen

2013 EDITION

Transferred to Digital Printing, 2012
Composition by TNQ Books and Journals Pvt Ltd, India

Editorial Office:
Elsevier
1600 John F. Kennedy Blvd.
Suite 1800
Philadelphia, PA 19103-2899

International Standard Serial Number: 1535-1513
International Standard Book Number: 978-1-4557-7287-2

Printed and bound by CPI Group (UK) Ltd, Croydon, CR0 4YY

Transferred to digital print 2012

Editorial Board

Table of Contents

Journals Represented

Journals represented in this YEAR BOOK are listed below.

Aesthetic Plastic Surgery
Aesthetic Surgery Journal
American Journal of Rhinology & Allergy
American Journal of Surgery
Annals of Plastic Surgery
Annals of Surgery
Annals of Surgical Oncology
Archives of Facial Plastic Surgery
Arthroscopy
Burns
Childs Nervous System
Cleft Palate-Craniofacial Journal
Clinical Orthopaedics and Related Research
Clinical Radiology
Cornea
Dermatologic Surgery
European Journal of Plastic Surgery
European Journal of Surgical Oncology
Head & Neck
Injury
Journal of Bone and Joint Surgery (American)
Journal of Bone and Joint Surgery (British)
Journal of Burn Care & Research
Journal of Cranio-Maxillo-Facial Surgery
Journal of Drugs in Dermatology
Journal of Hand Surgery
Journal of Plastic, Reconstructive & Aesthetic Surgery
Journal of Reconstructive Microsurgery
Journal of the American College of Surgeons
Journal of the European Academy of Dermatology & Venereology
Journal of Ultrasound in Medicine
Journal of Vascular Surgery
Laryngoscope
Microsurgery
New England Journal of Medicine
Ournal of Oral and Maxillofacial Surgery
Pediatric Dermatology
Plastic and Reconstructive Surgery

STANDARD ABBREVIATIONS

The following terms are abbreviated in this edition: acquired immunodeficiency syndrome (AIDS), cardiopulmonary resuscitation (CPR), central nervous system (CNS), cerebrospinal fluid (CSF), computed tomography (CT), deoxyribonucleic acid (DNA), electrocardiography (ECG), health maintenance organization (HMO), human immunodeficiency virus (HIV), intensive care unit (ICU), intramuscular

(IM), intravenous (IV), magnetic resonance (MR) imaging (MRI), ribonucleic acid (RNA), ultrasound (US), and ultraviolet (UV).

Introduction

This is the fifth year in which the YEAR BOOK OF PLASTIC AND AESTHETIC SURGERY has been published in both electronic and hard-copy formats. In the near future, it seems very likely that dual formats for the YEAR BOOK will be discontinued due to the diminishing number of subscriptions for hard-copy versions of virtually all of the annual YEAR BOOKS, including the YEAR BOOK OF PLASTIC AND AESTHETIC SURGERY. We hope plastic surgeons continue to find and read the commentaries and abstracts of the most essential articles in our field.

Once again, we have had several changes in the associate editorial staff. Dr James Boehmler of the Ohio State University School of Medicine (OSU) has joined our associate editor staff, replacing Dr Robert Ruberg, who has officially "retired" from Ohio State University. In keeping with his value to the OSU School of Medicine, Dr Ruberg has assumed a position as a Special Assistant to the Dean of the School of Medicine for Accreditation. We are very grateful to Dr Ruberg for mentoring Dr Boehmler this year, and for his willingness and commitment to continue to submit several selections and critiques.

I am grateful for the many fine contributions in years past from Dr Geoffrey Gurtner, who left our associate editorial staff just prior to the onset of this year's efforts. His contributions added immeasurably to the value of the YEAR BOOK OF PLASTIC AND AESTHETIC SURGERY. I am indebted to Dr David Smith Jr and Dr Karol Gutkowski for their superb and continuing efforts in past years, but especially for their hard work this year. They have done yeoman's work in combing the plastic surgical literature as well as the literature of related disciplines to select worthwhile articles to review and present to our readership. I would be remiss if I did not acknowledge the contributions of Dr Amanda Grosman.

I would also like to acknowledge the contributions of two of my plastic surgical colleagues from the University of California San Diego: Drs Ralph Holmes and Mayer Tennenhaus.

Thanks to Joanne Husovski, Senior Clinics Editor with Elsevier, who aided and assisted our effort this year. Her reminders were most helpful in encouraging many of the associate editors to meet and in several instances exceed their goals for selections.

As in the past, associate editors have been free to submit selections in several different areas beyond those to which they had been assigned. Not infrequently, this has resulted in having more than one editor review and critique the same selection, potentially providing the reader with differing viewpoints on the same article. We believe these differing viewpoints add value to the YEAR BOOK.

I call the reader's attention to several noteworthy articles:

(1) From Dr Ruberg comes Tissue transfer in the morbidly obese
(2) From Dr Smith: Exploring the application of stem cells in tendon repair and regeneration

(3) From Dr Miller comes Tissue-engineered breast reconstruction: Bridging the gap toward large-volume tissue engineering in humans
(4) Also from Miller: An update on facial transplantation cases performed between 2005 and 2010

Stephen H. Miller, MD, MPH

1 Congenital

Auricular Deformities

A prospective study on non-surgical correction of protruding ears: The importance of early treatment
van Wijk MP, Breugem CC, Kon M (Wilhelmina Children's Hosp Univ Med Ctr Utrecht, The Netherlands)
J Plast Reconstr Aesthet Surg 65:54-60, 2012

Objectives.—Splinting is an elegant method to correct ear deformities in the newborn. However evidence is lacking on the relation between age and efficacy and duration of the treatment. We prospectively studied these questions on protruding ears in 132 babies.

Methods.—A splint in the scaphal hollow was used in combination with tape (Earbuddies®). Treatment continued until the desired shape persisted. Results were judged from photographs and mastoid-helical distance was measured.

Results.—In 132 babies 209 ears were treated. Twenty-four patients had no follow-up, 27 stopped therapy for skin irritation and fixation problems. In the remaining patients results were good in 28%, fair in 36%, poor in 36%. Efficacy deteriorates with age; with fair or good results in 66.7% if therapy started before the sixth week. Older children needed to be splinted longer. The anti-helical fold was easier corrected than a deep concha (correction in 69.8% versus 26.8%).

Conclusions.—Considering splinting therapy for protruding ears, a reasonable chance of success can only be offered to parents of children up to six weeks of age. It is favorable if the deformity is mainly due to a flat anti-helix (Fig 1).

▶ This is an interesting prospective report from the Netherlands regarding the nonsurgical correction of protruding ears. The authors point to a large body of anecdotal evidence in the literature suggesting that the results of such therapy are good but note the lack of substantiation and the many questions remaining in assessing the effectiveness of this approach. Overall, the results reported by these authors are not overwhelmingly positive; only 60% of their patients completed treatment and/or were available for follow-up; in 36% of those who completed the treatment, the outcome was poor. Nonetheless, the study provides some useful information: treatment must begin early, preferably before

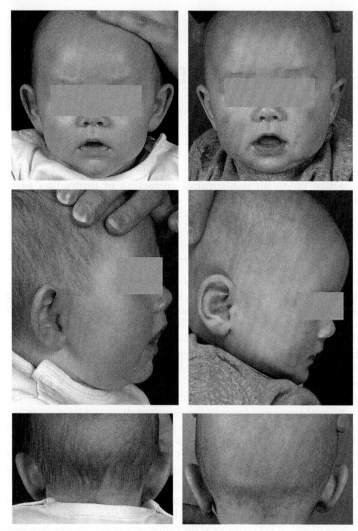

FIGURE 1.—a—f. left: protruding ear due to a flat antihelix and deep concha in a 10 weeks old boy. right: same boy after 12 weeks of splinting therapy. Good result. (Reprinted from van Wijk MP, Breugem CC, Kon M. A prospective study on non-surgical correction of protruding ears: the importance of early treatment. *J Plast Reconstr Aesthet Surg.* 2012;65:54-60, Copyright 2012, with permission from British Association of Plastic, Reconstructive and Aesthetic Surgeons.)

6 weeks of age and likely even earlier than that; best results are achieved when the problem was related to a flattened antihelical fold than when the problem was due to a deep concha; and finally, treatment can be expected to continue for at least 10 weeks. Perhaps, as discussed by Byrd et al,[1] the correction of a deep concha, because of its stiffer cartilage, requires more pressure, using a more rigid splint, to correct than does the less stiff antihelical fold. Data regarding changes in the mastoid-helical rim distance is difficult to assess

because normative changes in this distance in growing children have not been well established.

S. H. Miller, MD

Reference

1. Byrd HS, Langevin CJ, Ghidoni LA. Ear molding in newborn infants with auricular deformities. *Plast Reconstr Surg.* 2010;126:1191-2000.

A 2-Stage Ear Reconstruction for Microtia
Jiang H, Pan B, Zhao Y, et al (Plastic Surgery Hosp, Beijing, China)
Arch Facial Plast Surg 13:162-166, 2011

Objective.—To introduce our 2-stage reconstruction of microtia method, which results in a natural-looking contour of the reconstructed ears, one of the most demanding challenges in facial plastic surgery.

Methods.—In the first stage, the 3-dimensional cartilage framework is fabricated. The skin flap and retroauricular fascial flap are elevated in the mastoid area. Then the framework is wrapped by the fascial flap from behind and covered by the skin flap from front. In the second stage the crus, the tragus, and the conchal cavity are reconstructed. So almost all of the fine structures of ear are reconstructed.

Results.—Sixty-eight patients ranging in age from 5 to 17 years had their ears reconstructed using our 2-stage method from January 1, 2006, to December 31, 2008. Forty-eight patients were boys, and 20 were girls. Unilateral microtia was present in 66 patients and bilateral microtia was present in 2 patients. The reconstructed ears had a 3-dimensional configuration, and the cranioauricular angle of the reconstructed ears was similar to that of the contralateral ear.

Conclusions.—Two-stage ear reconstruction is a simple and promising method for microtia. Furthermore, the complications are rare.

▶ The authors present a 3-year series of 68 ear reconstructions using a 2-stage technique. In stage 1 the cartilage framework is fabricated from costal cartilages 6, 7, and 8. The anterior surface is covered by an anteriorly based skin flap and the postauricular surface by a posteriorly based fascial flap lined with a skin graft from the chest skin overlying the costal graft site. The ear lobe is also repositioned. In stage 2 the helical crus, tragus, and concha are created, utilizing the vestigial remnant ear. Excellent results are illustrated with photographs.

This article represents an evolution of experience and techniques by the authors that can be appreciated by reading their previous publications. They have discontinued the use of tissue expansion, thus reducing the number of stages from 3 to 2. They have created a classification of ear lobe position along with surgical modifications for each type. Their use of the vestigial remnant ear for reconstruction, rather than being discarded, is creative. And their use of cartilage removed to create the scapha to define the antihelix is a novel contribution. The result of their evolution, culminating in this current article, is a remarkable achievement of outstanding results in 2 surgeries.

R. Holmes, MD

Cleft Lip and Palate

Submucous Cleft Palate and Velopharyngeal Insufficiency: Comparison of Speech Outcomes Using Three Operative Techniques by One Surgeon
Sullivan SR, Vasudavan S, Marrinan EM, et al (Children's Hosp, Boston, MA; State Univ of New York, Syracuse)
Cleft Palate Craniofac J 48:561-570, 2011

Objective.—Our purpose was to compare speech outcomes among three primary procedures for symptomatic submucous cleft palate (SMCP): two-flap palatoplasty with muscular retropositioning, double-opposing Z-palatoplasty, or pharyngeal flap.

Design.—Retrospective review.

Setting.—Tertiary hospital.

Patients, Participants.—All children with SMCP treated by the senior author between 1984 and 2008.

Interventions.—One of three primary procedures: two-flap palatoplasty with muscular retropositioning, double-opposing Z-palatoplasty, or pharyngeal flap.

Main Outcome Measures.—Speech outcome and need for a secondary operation were analyzed among procedures. Success was defined as normal or borderline competent velopharyngeal function. Failure was defined as persistent borderline insufficiency or velopharyngeal insufficiency with recommendation for a secondary operation.

Results.—We identified 58 patients with SMCP who were treated for velopharyngeal insufficiency. We found significant differences in median age at operation among the procedures ($p < .001$). Two-flap palatoplasty with muscular retropositioning (n = 24), double-opposing Z-palatoplasty (n = 19), and pharyngeal flap (n = 15) were performed at a median of 2.5, 3.6, and 9.5 years, respectively. There were significant differences in success among procedures ($p = .018$). Normal or borderline competent function was achieved in 6/20 (30%) patients who underwent two-flap palatoplasty, 10/15 (67%) following double-opposing Z-palatoplasty, and 11/12 (92%) following pharyngeal flap. Among patients treated with palatoplasty, success was independent of age at operation ($p = .16$).

Conclusions.—Double-opposing Z-palatoplasty is more effective than two-flap palatoplasty with muscular retropositioning. For children older than 4 years, primary pharyngeal flap is also highly successful but equally so as a secondary operation and can be reserved, if necessary, following double-opposing Z-palatoplasty.

▶ This article is appealing in that it compares the speech outcomes of children with submucous cleft palate treated with different surgical techniques performed by a single surgeon. The perpetual challenge with assessing outcomes in the treatment of patients with clefts is to control as many of the variables (timing, surgeon, cleft type, standardized outcome tool) so the effect of any given intervention can be determined. It has been demonstrated that comparing different techniques performed by a single surgeon is significantly more valuable than comparing different techniques by different surgeons in the treatment of cleft palate. The difficulty with interpreting the data presented in this article is that there is no standard timing established for the treatment of submucous cleft palate, the median ages are significantly different between treatment groups, and the decision to perform a certain procedure over another was based on age or the perceived effectiveness of the chosen technique. Despite these confounding variables, the authors did find significant differences in the speech outcomes in the patients treated with different techniques.

The evolution of the featured author's treatment protocol is summarized in the article. Early in this author's career, patients under 5 years of age were treated with a 2-flap palatoplasty (median age 2.5 years). Because of dissatisfaction with the results of the 2-flap palatoplasty, in 1997 the author started to perform a double-opposing Z-palatoplasty, as described by Furlow, in patients under age 5 (median age 3.6 years). Patients aged 5 years or older who were able to participate in videofluoroscopy were treated with a primary pharyngeal flap (median age 9.5 years). The differences in the median ages between the treatment groups were statistically significant ($P < .001$). Speech outcomes were subjectively and objectively based on the perceptual assessment of structurally correctable variables of resonance (hypernasality or hyponasality), intraoral pressure, and nasal emission (on mirror examination), and whether the patients (or their families) reported a personal or social problem because of their speech. Speech outcomes were recorded by multiple speech pathologists without any evaluation of interrater variability.

According to the author's definition of successful speech outcomes, only 30% of the 2-flap palatoplasty group had a successful outcome after primary repair and a second procedure was recommended in 70% of patients. In the Z-plasty group, 67% of the patients had a successful primary operation, and secondary pharyngeal flap was recommended in 33% of patients. Although the authors report that there was no difference in the median age at palatoplasty and the need for secondary surgery, these findings were not statistically significant. In the pharyngeal flap group, 92% of the patients had a successful operative outcome. The potential morbidity of hyponasality and sleep apnea after pharyngeal flap make this a less popular treatment option than a functional palate repair.

The authors recommend the Furlow Z-palatoplasty over the 2-flap palatoplasty for primary repair of submucous cleft palate in children under 4 years and use of the pharyngeal flap as a secondary option.

A. Gosman, MD

Academic Achievement in Individuals With Cleft: A Population-Based Register Study

Persson M, Becker M, Svensson H (Bristol Dental School, UK; Malmö Univ Hosp, Sweden; Univ of Lund, Malmö, Sweden)
Cleft Palate-Craniofac J 49:153-159, 2012

Objective.—The focus of this study was to determine whether there were any significant differences in academic achievement between students with a cleft and the general population of Swedish students at the typical time of graduation from compulsory school (usually 16 years of age).

Design.—A retrospective population-based study. Data were obtained from the Swedish Medical Birth Register for the years 1973 through 1986 and were linked to the Swedish School—Grade Register.

Participants.—A total of 511 individuals with cleft palate (CP), 651 individuals with cleft lip (CL), and 830 individuals with cleft lip and palate (CLP) were compared with a control group consisting of 1,249,404 individuals.

Main Outcome Measures.—(1) Not receiving school leaving certificate; (2) odds of receiving lowest grade and reduced odds of receiving a high grade in the following subjects: (a) Mathematics, (b) English, (c) Swedish, (d) Physical Education, and (e) grade point average (GPA).

Results.—The group with cleft had higher odds of not receiving leaving certificates in comparison with the general population. They also had higher odds of receiving the lowest grade and/or reduced odds of receiving a high grade in the subjects analyzed together, with strong evidence of lower GPA in comparison with the general population. Individuals with CP were affected the most, followed by individuals with CLP; least affected were individuals with CL.

Conclusion.—This study clearly indicates that adolescents with cleft lip and/or palate in Sweden experience significant deficits in their educational achievements in compulsory school.

▶ The authors present a large retrospective study evaluating the academic achievement of students with clefts in Sweden. The authors were able to utilize cross-linked data from the Swedish Medical Birth Register (MBR), the Registrar of Congenital Malformations, and the Swedish School-Grade Register for 1992 individuals born with a cleft between 1973 and 1986. This population-based study demonstrates that children with clefts experience significant deficits in academic achievement compared with the general population, with the cleft palate group performing the worst (Fig 1 in the original article). There is some question about the possible inclusion of children with syndromes that may not have had updated information in the Register; the authors identify 229 of these cases that they excluded, but there may have been more that were not recognized. Overall, this is an important study that contributes to our acknowledgment of significant academic achievement deficits in this population and should be a springboard for further analysis of the underlying factors contributing to this phenomenon. Further research into the cognitive, social, and health-related factors that contribute to poor academic outcomes in children with clefts are necessary to understand and address the personal and societal impact.

A. Gosman, MD

Pharyngeal flap versus sphincter pharyngoplasty for the treatment of velopharyngeal insufficiency: A meta-analysis

Collins J, Cheung K, Farrokhyar F, et al (McMaster Univ, Hamilton, Ontario, Canada)
J Plast Reconstr Aesthet Surg 65:864-868, 2012

Background.—Velopharyngeal insufficiency (VPI) has been reported in 5–20% of patients following cleft palate repair. Since VPI can limit communication, determining which operative procedure leads to the greatest improvement is of utmost importance. Since there is no consensus, this meta-analysis aims to determine which procedure results in the most significant resolution of VPI.

Methods.—Two independent assessors undertook a literature review for articles that compare procedures aimed at treating VPI. Study quality was determined using validated scales. Level of agreement was assessed using intra-class coalition coefficient analysis. The heterogeneity between studies was evaluated using I^2 and Cochran's Q-statistic. Random effect model analysis and forest plots were used to report a pooled odds ratio (OR) and 95% confidence intervals (CI) for treatment effect. A p-value of 0.05 was considered for statistical significance.

Results.—Two randomised controlled trials (RCTs) comparing pharyngeal flap to sphincter pharyngoplasty were obtained. A total of 133 patients were included, with follow-ups at 3–4 months. The pooled OR was determined to be 2.95 (95% CI: 0.66–13.23) in favour of the pharyngeal flap.

Conclusions.—Based on these RCTs, which currently compose the highest quality data that compares pharyngeal flap versus pharyngoplasty, the pooled treatment effect suggests a possible trend favouring pharyngeal flap.

▶ This article examines an important issue that needs to be resolved, although the results of the meta-analysis, based on an analysis of the pooled data from 2 randomized controlled trials (RCT) reported by these authors, seem to favor the use of a superiorly based pharyngeal flap rather than a sphincter-based pharyngoplasty. However, even the 2 RCTs, 1 being multi-institutional and 1 being from a single institution, are somewhat flawed in their methodological designs. Clearly a large RCT multi-institutional study with strict guidelines for inclusion or exclusion, postoperative follow-up, and adequate numbers of patients in each of the arms of the study would be most welcome to definitively answer which of the 2 techniques is better for ameliorating velopharyngeal incompetence.

S. H. Miller, MD

Cranio-Maxillo-Facial

Visual field loss in children with craniosynostosis

Liasis A, Walters B, Thompson D, et al (Great Ormond St Hosp for Children, London, UK)
Childs Nerv Syst 27:1289-1296, 2011

Aims.—To identify visual field deficits in a group of children with syndromic craniosynostosis.

Methods.—Kinetic visual field examination and visual evoked potentials (VEPs) were recorded in 16 children with syndromic craniosynostosis as part of their ophthalmic evaluation. VEPs were analyzed for inter-hemispheric asymmetries and component amplitude and latency, while visual fields were analyzed both qualitatively and quantitatively.

Results.—All children with craniosynostosis were found to have visual field deficits compared to controls. In the Crouzon group, deficits tended to involve the nasal field, while infero-nasal field deficits were the most consistent finding in children with Apert syndrome. Children with Pfeiffer's demonstrated the greatest deficits, with severe constrictions affecting the whole visual field. VEPs were asymmetrical in four cases while the P100 component was subnormal in ten of the 16 patients for either amplitude and/or latency.

Conclusion.—Although we may speculate about the mechanisms that cause visual field deficits, we currently are unable to explain the reason for the differing types and extent of visual field loss in the different syndromic groups. We can conclude that the visual field deficits do indicate previous or ongoing visual dysfunction that cannot be monitored employing central vision tests alone.

▶ This is an interesting contribution to the literature pertaining to visual impairment in children with syndromic craniosynostosis. Changes in the visual field are not routinely evaluated or monitored in children with craniosynostosis, and the assessment of their visual function has traditionally been based on central vision tests and the measurement of visual acuity. This article shows that there are significant visual field changes in these patients, and, based on these findings, surgeons should consider the evaluation and monitoring of visual field impairment in patients treated for craniosynostosis. Although the mechanism of visual field impairment is not clear and could be multifactorial, these findings are important and worthy of further study. Early visual field assessment and monitoring in patients with craniosynostosis would be an important step toward understanding the natural progression and possible avoidance of their visual impairment.

A. Gosman, MD

Comparison of mandibular vertical growth in hemifacial microsomia patients treated with early distraction or not treated: Follow up till the completion of growth

Meazzini MC, Mazzoleni F, Bozzetti A, et al (Univ of Milano-Bicocca, Monza, Italy; et al)

J Cranio-Maxillo-Fac Surg 40:105-111, 2012

Aim.—Comparison of the long-term follow-up until the completion of growth of two homogeneous samples of children affected by hemifacial microsomia (HFM), one treated by mandibular distraction osteogenesis (DO) in the deciduous or early mixed dentition, the other not subjected to any treatment until adulthood.

Material.—Fourteen patients affected by vertically severe type I or II HFM were operated at an average age of 5.9 years with an average follow-up of 11.2 years. They were compared to a sample of eight patients who were never treated until the completion of growth.

Methods.—Mandibular vertical changes were measured on panoramic radiographs taken at different time points. Ratios between affected and non affected ramal heights were calculated and compared.

Results.—In the DO sample, after correction, mandibular vertical changes showed a gradual return of the asymmetry with growth in all patients. The ratio in the non treated sample was unchanged between the initial and the long term panoramic x-rays.

Conclusion.—The facial proportions of HFM patients are maintained, when not treated, throughout growth. The same proportions return to their original asymmetry after DO. Even though short term aesthetic and psychological advantages of distraction osteogenesis are well accepted, early surgery should only be applied after careful patient selection and honest clarification of the long term recurrence by genetically guided cranio-facial growth pattern (Fig 2).

▶ The authors present a compelling prospective comparison of the long-term growth patterns of 2 groups of children with hemifacial microsomia, one that has been treated with distraction osteogenesis and another that has not been treated. The patient groups were similar, and vertical lengthening of the ramus was achieved with distraction in the treatment group. The main outcome measure was the ratio of the ramus height on the affected versus the unaffected side. The authors report that after complete correction of the ratio during distraction, that 16% ± 17% of the vertical correction obtained by distraction was lost at the end of the first year and 75% ± 11% of the vertical correction was lost after 5 years. At the final follow-up after growth was completed (> 10 years after distraction) the ratio of ramus height was virtually unchanged from the predistraction ratio. This is well illustrated in Fig 2. The ratio of ramus height was also constant in the untreated group.

The authors were able to achieve significant vertical lengthening of the ramus with distraction osteogenesis, but the results were short lived, and the asymmetric ratios recurred when growth was complete. These patients may benefit

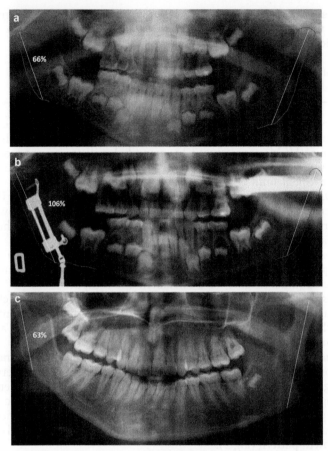

FIGURE 2.—a: Panoramic x-rays of a right type I HFM pre-distraction (T0) with a ratio between affected and non affected ramus of 66%; b: At end of distraction, right before the removal of the pins (Td); c: 13 years post distraction (Tlt) with a ratio between affected and non affected ramus of 63%. (Reprinted from Meazzini MC, Mazzoleni F, Bozzetti A, et al. Comparison of mandibular vertical growth in hemifacial microsomia patients treated with early distraction or not treated: follow up till the completion of growth. *J Cranio-Maxillo-Fac Surg*. 2012;40:105—111, with permission from European Association for Cranio-Maxillo-Facial Surgery.)

from the temporary symmetry achieved but will likely require additional surgery when they are mature. The authors postulate that there may be genetic input guiding the neuromuscular imbalance that rejects new musculo-skeletal geometry. However, the article does not include any assessments of actual ramus height measurements to evaluate how much the ramus actually grew after distraction and whether there was a growth restriction after surgery. It would be interesting to know the growth rate of the ramus after distraction and in relation to the growth rate of the unaffected side. The authors also do not discuss the advantages of mandibular distraction on the growth and incline of the maxilla on the affected side. Did mandibular distraction permit greater maxillary growth on the affected side? The need for definitive correction of the asymmetry at the age of maturity and what procedures were indicated or performed would provide additional information that would be helpful when counseling patients on the risks and benefits of early distraction ontogenesis during mixed dentition.

A. Gosman, MD

Changes in Frontal Morphology after Single-Stage Open Posterior—Middle Vault Expansion for Sagittal Craniosynostosis

Khechoyan D, Schook C, Birgfeld CB, et al (Seattle Children's Hosp, WA; Brigham Young Univ, Provo, UT)
Plast Reconstr Surg 129:504-516, 2012

Background.—There is controversy regarding whether the frontal bossing associated with sagittal synostosis requires direct surgical correction or spontaneously remodels after isolated posterior cranial expansion. The authors retrospectively measured changes in frontal bone morphology in patients with isolated sagittal synostosis 2 years after open posterior and midvault cranial expansion and compared these changes with those occurring in age-comparable healthy control groups.

Methods.—Forty-three patients age 1 year or younger (mean, 6 months) with sagittal synostosis underwent computed tomography scan digital analysis immediately after and 2 years after posterior—middle cranial vault expansion. Quantitative angular and linear measures were taken along the midsagittal and axial planes to capture both aspects of frontal bossing. The change in values over the 2 years were compared with healthy controls with normal computed tomography scans taken to rule out head trauma.

Results.—All measures indicative of frontal bossing decreased significantly from the time of posterior—middle vault expansion to 2 years postoperatively. Whereas the majority of patients at time of the operation had frontal bossing measures greater than two standard deviations outside the age-comparable control mean, almost all patients were within two standard deviations of the norm 2 years later. Lateral forehead bossing and anterior cranial growth was greater the older the patient was at the time of the operation, suggesting that the more time that passed before the operation, the more compensatory anterior fossa growth occurred. Central forehead position relative to the anterior cranial base was greatest in the younger patients at the time of operation, suggesting that a central forehead bulge was an early compensatory response to premature sagittal fusion.

Conclusions.—As a group, patients with sagittal synostosis start to normalize their forehead morphology within 2 years if an isolated posterior operation is performed at 1 year of age or younger, and this occurs by a combination of restriction of growth and reduction relative to patients without synostosis. This protocol decreases the risks of intraoperative positioning, forehead contour deformities, and two-stage operations.

Clinical Question/Level of Evidence.—Therapeutic, III.

▶ The authors in this study use a variety of axial and sagittal digital measurements of postoperative CT scans to assess the changes in frontal morphology after open posterior cranial expansion for sagittal craniosynostosis. Measurements from the immediate postoperative period and 2 years after surgery are compared with 2 different groups of normal healthy controls. The control group patients are different at the 2 time points and do not have consecutive scans, which is a limitation of the study.

The axial plane measurements differed with statistical significance from controls immediately after surgery but not at 2-year follow-up. Midsagittal plane measurements included a mean bossing angle that differed with near statistical significance at 2-year follow-up with an angle of 110 ± 4 degrees in the experimental group compared to 108 ± 4 degrees for the control ($P = .054$). The authors argued that this difference in the mean bossing angle was just outside statistical significance ($P < .05$) and then reevaluated the data according to "clinical frontal bossing," which they defined as being 2 standard deviations from the mean of the control group. Using this reinterpretation of the data, 85% of the patients at 2-year follow-up were within 2 standard deviations of the mean compared with 4% immediately after surgery.

Overall the authors present a more comprehensive method of performing digital measurements to analyze changes in frontal morphology after posterior cranial expansion than has been previously described. The results support the effectiveness of posterior vault expansion in reducing frontal bossing in sagittal craniosynostosis. Comparison with a consecutive control group and with another experimental group that undergoes anterior cranial vault remodeling would be additive.

A. Gosman, MD

Vascular Malformations

A Prospective Self-Controlled Phase II Study of Imiquimod 5% Cream in the Treatment of Infantile Hemangioma

Jiang CH, Hu XJ, Ma G, et al (Shanghai Jiaotong Univ, China)
Pediatr Dermatol 28:259-266, 2011

Imiquimod has been reported to be efficacious in the topical treatment of uncomplicated infantile hemangiomas (IH). However, due to the natural tendency of IH to involute spontaneously, prior uncontrolled efficacy and safety studies have been called into question. We conducted a prospective self-controlled phase II study of imiquimod initially applied to uncomplicated, proliferative superficial or mixed IHs treating half of each IH once every other night for 16 weeks, leaving the other half untreated. After 16 weeks, an independent dermatologist evaluated the color, area, and volume of each half of the hemangioma. Of the 44 patients treated, the total effective rate was 80% ($n = 35$), with an overall resolution rated as excellent or good rate in 39% of lesions ($n = 17/44$). The relapse rate was

2% (*n* = 1). Side effects were noted in 61% (*n* = 27) including erythema or/and edema (*n* = 16%, 7), local itching (*n* = 7%, 3), peeling (*n* = 7%, 3), erosion (*n* = 5%, 2), crusting (*n* = 55%, 24), ulceration (*n* = 9%, 4), and scarring (*n* = 5%, 2). Some patients had two or more side effects. Most were judged to be mild to moderate and did not result in treatment being interrupted. Crusting or ulceration was noted to cause post-treatment skin reactions, such as texture change, whereas cases without crusting involuted to almost normal skin. No local infection or systemic reaction was observed. The difference in effective rate and side effect incidence between superficial and mixed IH was not statistically significant. Imiquimod 5% cream can be an effective and safe treatment option for superficial mixed IH in which the superficial component predominates. The recurrence rate is low, but local reactions including crusting can develop and result in post-treatment skin changes.

▶ This prospective study looks at the effect of topical imiquimod 5% (Aldara) on infantile hemangiomas. Imiquimod is applied to half of the lesion, and the other half of the lesion acts as the control. Of the 44 patients, 6.8% (n = 3) of the lesions resolved and 39% (n = 17) of the lesions either resolved or had a good or excellent response to treatment. The incidence of side effects was significant in 61% of patient with crusting being the most common (55%). Of the 25 patients who had moderate to excellent responses, 17 experienced crusting, and 65% (n = 11) had posttreatment skin reactions, including scarring or pigment or texture change. This is a significant complication rate in the best responders. The treatment was continued for 16 weeks, but rest periods were given "to manage side effects as needed," although the duration of the rest periods and the patients who required rest are not identified, nor is their eventual outcome.

If more than half of the patients who responded will have permanent skin changes, it is difficult to justify treatment with imiquimod 5% if skin changes are avoided by nontreatment and allowing the lesion to involute.

A. Gosman, MD

Miscellaneous

Closure of Large Myelomeningocele by Lumbar Artery Perforator Flaps
El-Sabbagh AH, Zidan AS (Mansoura Univ Hosp, Dakahlia, Egypt)
J Reconstr Microsurg 27:287-294, 2011

Myelomeningocele is the most complex congenital malformation of the central nervous system that is compatible with life. Different closure techniques are available for defect reconstruction, but wound healing and tension-free closure of the skin in the midline remain major considerations in large myelomeningoceles. In this study, bilateral lumbar artery perforator flaps were used for closure of large myelomeningocele defects. Fifteen infants and neonates with large myelomeningocele defects were enrolled in the study. The lumbar artery perforator flaps were elevated bilaterally or unilaterally and advanced toward the midline without tension and were

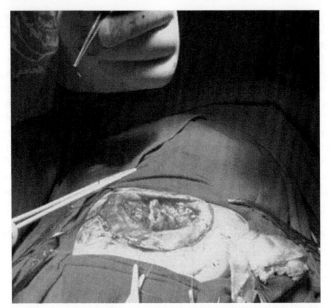

FIGURE 1.—Closure of neural tube. (Reprinted from El-Sabbagh AH, Zidan AS. Closure of large myelomeningocele by lumbar artery perforator flaps. *J Reconstr Microsurg.* 2011;27:287-293, with permission from Thieme Medical Publishers, Inc.)

sutured together. Most of the flaps healed without any major complication. The lumbar artery perforator flaps as is an effective method for closure of large myelomeningocele defects (Fig 1).

▶ Myelomeningocele repair can be a challenge to repair, and traditional repairs frequently involve large myocutaneous flaps. This article is an excellent example of performing perforator flap surgery without the need for microsurgery. It also highlights the knowledge that flaps that were once considered "random" can frequently be designed and planned as an axial pattern flap with a source vessel. By creating transposition flaps with axial blood supply, a surgeon can have a logical stepwise plan to perform 1 or (if needed) 2 flaps to close some relatively large defects (Fig 1). Also, by isolating the flap on the lumbar perforators, the latissimus muscle is preserved and remains completely functional, which will likely have long-term rehabilitation advantages. Care needs to be taken in raising these flaps so that there is adequate dissection and freeing of the pedicle to prevent kinking of the vascular supply as it is rotated into position.

J. Boehmler, MD

2 Neoplastic, Inflammatory and Degenerative Conditions

Facial Nerve Paralysis

Pectoralis minor muscle transfer for unilateral facial palsy reanimation: An experience of 35 years and 637 cases

Harrison DH, Grobbelaar AO (Suite 2, London, UK; Royal Free Hosp, London, UK)

J Plast Reconstr Aesthet Surg 65:845-850, 2012

Background.—Free functional muscle transfers are often the treatment of choice for facial reanimation. We describe our experience with 637 cases over a 35-year period.

Methods.—Data was collected prospectively on all case undergoing functional muscle transfer for unilateral facial paralysis. Results were judged by the operating surgeon and an Independent panel of four observers.

Results.—354 patients had an excellent result as judged by the surgeon. An independent panel rated patients to have a significant change pre- and post-operatively comparing their Hay's scores ($p < 0.001$, t-test). 27.2% of patients required revisional procedures. 13.3% of patients developed late onset tightness of the transferred muscle.

Conclusions.—Facial reanimation with functional muscle transfers is a complex procedure and provides a significant improvement for the patient to display humour and emotion.

▶ Free functional muscle transfers are often the treatment of choice for facial reanimation. The authors describe their experience with 637 cases over a 35-year period. This is an extraordinary series and worth reviewing by anyone interested in or doing this surgery. Unfortunately, there is not as much in-depth information as desired. Nevertheless, Douglas Harrison has been interested in this surgery throughout his career, and the exceptional quality of the outcomes is a testament to this dedication.

D. J. Smith, Jr, MD

Head and Neck Reconstruction

The Spiral Flap for Nasal Alar Reconstruction: Our Experience with 63 Patients
Mahlberg MJ, Leach BC, Cook J (Med Univ of South Carolina, Charleston)
Dermatol Surg 38:373-380, 2012

Objective.—To describe our patient selection, design, execution, and results with the spiral flap for distal nasal surgical defects after Mohs micrographic surgery.

Materials and Methods.—We performed a retrospective analysis of all spiral flaps performed over a 5-year period. Sixty-three patients were identified, and charts and photographs were examined. Surgical defects were classified according to alar location. All follow-up encounters were reviewed to assess for complications and need for revisionary procedures. Intraoperative photographs were taken of representative cases to describe the surgical technique.

Results.—Sixty-three patients on whom the spiral flap was performed were identified over a 5-year period. The flap was used to successfully reconstruct alar defects ranging in size from 5 to 15 mm in diameter. No persistent complications were noted.

Conclusion.—The spiral flap is a reproducible, one-stage flap for small to medium-sized defects of the nasal ala and alar groove that consistently produces topographic restoration with minimal risk of aesthetic or functional complication (Fig 2).

▶ Robbing Peter to pay Paul is a standard mantra in reconstructive surgery, and nowhere else is this truer than in the case of the nose. Because of dense, thick tip and alar skin, primary repair is generally not feasible without significant distortion of the nasal structures. Most small- to medium-sized repairs of tip and alar defects involve bringing tissue from the middle or upper nose (or cheek) into the defect. Alar reconstruction can be especially problematic because of the concave nature of the alar groove and the convexity of the ala itself. This article is a nice description and series of a spiral flap used for alar reconstructions of defects from 5 to 15 mm. They describe the origins of the spiral form (Archimedes wrote about them in 225 BC in On Spirals), and how the logarithmic pattern is potentially a 1-stage reconstructive option. In reviewing their photos, I'm not quite convinced that they actually create a full spiral, as the design generally makes it from 180° to 270° around the defect (Fig 2). In reality, this is a rotation flap with the distal tip tucked in on itself to help reestablish the alar crease. Regardless of the designation, they show good consistent results. The obvious concern would be for the potential of nasal tip elevation, which they state was not a long-term issue. I also felt that some of the patients may have had a

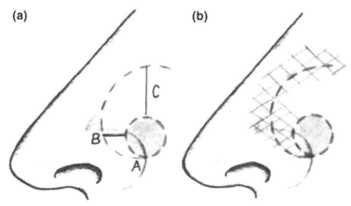

FIGURE 2.—Design elements of spiral flap. Three important points should be considered in designing a spiral flap that will satisfy the reconstructive requirements of the surgical defect. (a) Point A is the point at which the flap originates from the wound edge. Point B designates the anterior projection of the spiral that will approximate the vertical height of the wound. Point C designates the vertical height and thus the angle of curvature of the spiral. (b) Areas that should be undermined to provide flap mobility while maintaining the myocutaneous pedicle. (Reprinted from Mahlberg MJ, Leach BC, Cook J. The spiral flap for nasal alar reconstruction: our experience with 63 patients. *Dermatol Surg.* 2012;38:373-380, with permission from Wiley & Sons, Inc.)

small cone or "spiral" of cheek skin brought onto the nasal sidewall, which could create some asymmetry but is difficult to assess because only the operated side was shown in the photos.

J. Boehmler, MD

Perforator-Based Myocutaneous Pedicle Flap for Reconstruction of a Large Defect of the Posterior Ear

Vergilis-Kalner IJ, Goldberg LH, Landau JM, et al (UMDNJ - Robert Wood Johnson Med School, NJ; Derm Surgery Associates, Houston, TX)
Dermatol Surg 38:932-936, 2012

Background.—The methods of repair used for defects of the posterior surface of the ear after tumor excision include second intention healing, simple linear closures, and full- or split-thickness skin grafts if the perichondrium and soft tissue are intact. If cartilage is exposed, local flaps are needed because grafts are unlikely to survive if the perichondrum is not intact. Coverage using a graft or flap is associated with less pain, minimal contraction with wound healing, and less risk of chondritis. Many type of flaps can be used. A case was reported in which a posterior auricular artery-n-based myocutaneous pedicle flap (MPF) was used successfully to reconstruct a large defect of the posterior ear with exposed cartilage.

Case Report.—Man, 77, had a 4.1-cm by 2.2-cm basal cell carcinoma on the posterior surface of his right ear removed through Mohs micrographic surgery, producing a 7.4-cm by 2.7-cm defect on the posterior ear with exposed cartilage. A one-stage reconstruction using readily available, hairless, well-vascularized donor skin from the superior lateral neck was undertaken. A template the size of the defect was cut out and used to outline and position the flap to be transferred. The flap was long enough to avoid excessive tension during suturing and wide enough to ensure adequate blood supply and allow for rotation without strangulation and restriction of its blood supply. Lidocaine 0.5% with epinephrine (1:200,000) was used to tumesce the skin of the donor site. The area was undermined but remained attached to the defect by the myocutaneous pedicle. After sufficient dissection and mobilization of the flap in the superficial subcutaneous plane, it was elevated, rotated 180°, and transposed into the defect, with interrupted 4-0 Ethilon sutures used to establish placement. Wound edges were averted during suturing to produce a smooth epidermal surface. The secondary defect was closed side to side as a primary linear closure. A pressure bandage was applied for 2 days, then traditional daily wound care was instituted. The flap healed well and provided satisfactory esthetic results in both the donor and the ear site, with minimal distortion of the ear's anatomy.

Conclusions.—The technique used for this patient involved a single-stage posterior auricular artery-n-based transposition MPF that yielded good

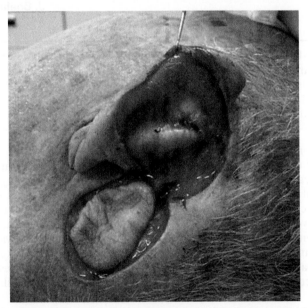

FIGURE 3.—The entire transposition flap was dissected and mobilized in the superficial subcutaneous plane. (Reprinted from Vergilis-Kalner IJ, Goldberg LH, Landau JM, et al. Perforator-based myocutaneous pedicle flap for reconstruction of a large defect of the posterior ear. *Dermatol Surg.* 2012;38:932-936, with permission from the American Society for Dermatologic Surgery, Inc.)

restoration of a large defect on the posterior ear. The site could not be left to heal by second intention, could not be closed primarily, and would not be sufficiently covered by a full-thickness skin graft, whose blood supply would likely be inadequate. The strong vascular supply of the MPF used

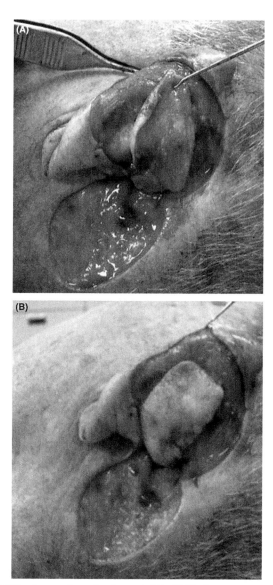

FIGURE 4.—(A) The flap was elevated and rotated 180°. (B) The flap was transposed into the defect. (Reprinted from Vergilis-Kalner IJ, Goldberg LH, Landau JM, et al. Perforator-based myocutaneous pedicle flap for reconstruction of a large defect of the posterior ear. *Dermatol Surg.* 2012;38:932-936, with permission from John Wiley & Sons, Inc.)

ensured the viability of the flap, and the location of the donor site was sufficiently hidden to produce a satisfactory esthetic result (Figs 3 and 4).

▶ This article highlights a few differences between dermatologic surgeons and plastic surgeons. The first issue is how this case report describes the reconstruction. It is described as a perforator-based myocutaneous flap. The assumption with such a label would be to allow the reconstructive surgeon to bill for a myocutaneous flap of the head and neck, which would be a fairly high relative value unit option given the amount of work. Unfortunately, this is not a myocutaneous flap but rather a local tissue rearrangement or island pedicle flap at best (Figs 3 and 4). They describe the flap as preserving the perforators, but only inasmuch as they leave a subcutaneous pedicle "which should be made as wide as possible, so as not to strangulate the flap." When a flap is not skeletonized down to its axial blood supply, but rather a soft tissue bridge containing the blood supply, it cannot be considered a myocutaneous flap for current procedural terminology coding. Also, the flap is raised in the subcutaneous plane, which is not the definition of a myocutaneous flap. Technically, it is a nice repair for a difficult problem, but I do question their use of a pressure dressing, since the flap did develop distal necrosis, which could have been attributed to pressure or twisting of the subcutaneous pedicle.

J. Boehmler, MD

Extremity and Trunk Reconstruction

A reusable perforator-preserving gluteal artery-based rotation fasciocutaneous flap for pressure sore reconstruction
Lin P-Y, Kuo Y-R, Tsai Y-T (Kaohsiung Chang Gung Memorial Hosp, Taiwan)
Microsurgery 32:189-195, 2012

Background.—Perforator-based fasciocutaneous flaps for reconstructing pressure sores can achieve good functional results with acceptable donor site complications in the short-term. Recurrence is a difficult issue and a major concern in plastic surgery. In this study, we introduce a reusable perforator-preserving gluteal artery-based rotation flap for reconstruction of pressure sores, which can be also elevated from the same incision to accommodate pressure sore recurrence.

Methods.—The study included 23 men and 13 women with a mean age of 59.3 (range 24–89) years. There were 24 sacral ulcers, 11 ischial ulcers, and one trochanteric ulcer. The defects ranged in size from 4×3 to 12×10 cm^2. Thirty-six consecutive pressure sore patients underwent gluteal artery-based rotation flap reconstruction. An inferior gluteal artery-based rotation fasciocutaneous flap was raised, and the superior gluteal artery perforator was preserved in sacral sores; alternatively, a superior gluteal artery-based rotation fasciocutaneous flap was elevated, and the inferior gluteal artery perforator was identified and dissected in ischial ulcers.

Results.—The mean follow-up was 20.8 (range 0–30) months in this study. Complications included four cases of tip necrosis, three wound dehiscences, two recurrences reusing the same flap for pressure sore reconstruction, one seroma, and one patient who died on the fourth postoperative day. The complication rate was 20.8% for sacral ulcers, 54.5% for ischial wounds, and none for trochanteric ulcer. After secondary repair and reconstruction of the compromised wounds, all of the wounds healed uneventfully.

Conclusions.—The perforator-preserving gluteal artery-based rotation fasciocutaneous flap is a reliable, reusable flap that provides rich vascularity facilitating wound healing and accommodating the difficulties of pressure sore reconstruction (Fig 3).

▶ Recurrence is obviously the most troublesome issue when caring for patients with sacral and ischial pressure ulcers. Although there are a variety of flaps described to assist in closure, more attention has been paid recently to large rotation flaps because of their ability to be reelevated and rotated again in the unfortunate (but likely) case of ulcer recurrence. Although the idea of muscle preservation and perforator use is not new for gluteal flaps, this study shows a rational approach to perforator flap management of pressure ulcer patients. Sacral ulcers are treated with a large, inferiorly based gluteal flap with intramuscular dissection of the superior gluteal artery perforators (SGAP) to allow for rotation of the flap while leaving the inferior gluteal perforators (IGAP) intact for a dual blood supply (Fig 3). The roles are reversed for ischial ulcers, where the IGAP is dissected free from the muscle to allow for rotation. This technique is very useful for the initial surgery to maximize blood supply and minimize muscle sacrifice, but it does add to operative time, compared to a standard

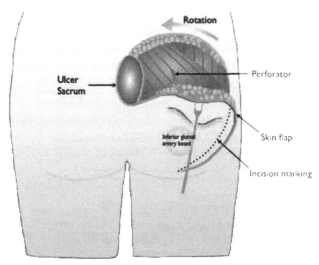

FIGURE 3.—Inferior gluteal artery-based rotation fasciocutaneous perforator flap with superior gluteal artery perforator preservation for the reconstruction of sacral sores. [Color figure can be viewed in the online issue, which is available at wileyonlinelibrary.com.] (Reprinted from Lin P-Y, Kuo Y-R, Tsai Y-T. A reusable perforator-preserving gluteal artery-based rotation fasciocutaneous flap for pressure sore reconstruction. *Microsurgery.* 2012;32:189-195, with permission from Wiley Periodicals, Inc.)

musculocutaneous flap. In the ambulatory patient, there is certainly benefit to this approach, but in the paraplegic or quadriplegic patient, it may not be as beneficial. They also do not discuss adequately the difficulty in reelevating the flap for recurrence, considering the perforator would now be encased in scar and easily injured during dissection. Of course, the flap would have been relatively delayed and would likely survive well if the additional perforator was sacrificed, assuming the other major blood supply was preserved. Regardless, their concept of large rotation flaps for reconstruction is well founded, given the recurrence rate of 21% for sacral wounds and 55% for ischial ulcers that required rerotation of the flap.

J. Boehmler, MD

Minimally Invasive Component Separation Results in Fewer Wound-Healing Complications than Open Component Separation for Large Ventral Hernia Repairs
Ghali S, Turza KC, Baumann DP, et al (The Univ of Texas MD Anderson Cancer Ctr, Houston)
J Am Coll Surg 214:981-989, 2012

Background.—Minimally invasive component separation (CS) with inlay bioprosthetic mesh (MICSIB) is a recently developed technique for abdominal wall reconstruction that preserves the rectus abdominis perforators and minimizes subcutaneous dead space using limited-access tunneled incisions. We hypothesized that MICSIB would result in better surgical outcomes than conventional open CS.

Study Design.—All consecutive patients who underwent CS (open or minimally invasive) with inlay bioprosthetic mesh for ventral hernia repair from 2005 to 2010 were included in a retrospective analysis of prospectively collected data. Surgical outcomes, including wound-healing complications, hernia recurrences, and abdominal bulge/laxity rates, were compared between patient groups based on the type of CS repair, either MICSIB or open.

Results.—Fifty-seven patients who underwent MICSIB and 50 who underwent open CS were included. Mean follow-ups were 15.2 ± 7.7 months and 20.7 ± 14.3 months, respectively. Mean fascial defect size was significantly larger in the MICSIB group (405.4 ± 193.6 cm^2 vs 273.8 ± 186.8 cm^2; $p = 0.002$). The incidences of skin dehiscence (11% vs 28%; $p = 0.011$), all wound-healing complications (14% vs 32%; $p = 0.026$), abdominal wall laxity/bulge (4% vs 14%; $p = 0.056$), and hernia recurrence (4% vs 8%; $p = 0.3$) were lower in the MICSIB group than in the open CS group.

Conclusions.—MICSIB resulted in fewer wound-healing complications than did open CS used for complex abdominal wall reconstructions. These findings are likely attributable to the preservation of paramedian skin vascularity and reduction in subcutaneous dead space with MICSIB.

MICSIB should be considered for complex abdominal wall reconstructions, particularly in patients at increased risk of wound-healing complications.

▶ Since the introduction of component separation for ventral hernia repairs, several modifications have been created to increase the ability of primary closure of the fascia but also to limit the expected complications. Minimally Invasive Component Separation with Inlay Bioprosthetic Mesh (MICSIB) is a technique described by the authors in which significant subcutaneous undermining is limited, and preservation of the rectus abdominis skin perforators are preserved to supply the paramedian skin paddles. This is a large study comparing 2 cohorts, the MICSIB versus a standard Component Separation (CS) with inlay biopros-thetic mesh. The authors do a nice job showing a decreased complication rate with MICSIB, particularly with wound healing, despite having a large average hernia surface area. There were also trends toward fewer bulges and reoperations in the MICSIB group. The only data that are missing that would have been inter-esting are the operating times needed for both groups. It is suspected that the MICSIB requires more operating time, especially when first learning the tech-nique, but likely gets more efficient with time. Also, none of their patients had synthetic mesh placement (all were bioprosthetic). It would be likely that some of these patients would have been candidates for a newer generation, multiply synthetic mesh, which would be less costly than the large sheets of bio-prosthetic mesh utilized. It would be nice to see a cohort of patients undergoing MICSIB with synthetic mesh for comparison. Regardless, it is a worthwhile endeavor to perform component separation with an attempt at perforator preser-vation to limit skin breakdown, as long as the minimal invasive nature of the surgery still allows for a full component release, which it does seem to from their data and results.

J. Boehmler, MD

A Modified Free Muscle Transfer Technique to Effectively Treat Chronic and Persistent Calcaneal Osteomyelitis

Ghods M, Grabs R, Kersten C, et al (Hosp Ernst von Bergmann, Potsdam, Germany)
Ann Plast Surg 68:599-605, 2012

Objective.—Successful management of chronic calcaneal osteomyelitis presents a major challenge for the plastic and reconstructive surgeon, espe-cially in cases involving soft-tissue defects. This article describes a modi-fied free muscle transfer technique to effectively eradicate chronic and persistent calcaneal osteomyelitis.

Methods.—Between February 2009 and September 2009, 3 male patients with persistent calcaneal osteomyelitis were treated in our clinic. All 3 had purulent drainage for a minimum of 6 months and a maximum of 23 years. Multiple surgical debridements and vacuum-assisted closure had been used in the past, but the infection remained. We used a therapeutic protocol of repeated and radical surgical debridement with removal of nearly all cancellous bone and preservation of the cortical shell of the calcaneus. After the final debridement, the bone cavity was plugged by a free gracilis muscle flap from the contralateral side. A meshed split thickness skin graft was applied. Culture-specific antibiotics were administered for 2 weeks.

Results.—All flaps healed uneventfully except for a minor hematoma that was treated conservatively. All 3 patients were able to return to ambulatory status with regular foot apparel. At last follow-up evaluation, they had no clinical, laboratory, or radiologic signs of osteomyelitis.

Conclusion.—This modified free muscle transfer technique seems to be successful in managing chronic and persistent calcaneal osteomyelitis. Infected and healthy cancellous bone of the calcaneus is removed to eradicate all possible foci that maintain inflammation. The resulting bony defect after the aggressive surgical debridement is sufficiently filled with a well-vascularized muscle that ensures a good wound healing. We consider this method to be a promising treatment option, which needs to be supported by further cases (Figs 7 and 8).

▶ Osteomyelitis is difficult to treat, and calcaneal osteomyelitis is doubly tough. Given the weight-bearing nature of the calcaneus and the frequent medical comorbidities seen in patients who develop osteomyelitis (diabetes, tobacco abuse, peripheral vascular disease), lower extremity salvage of this patient population is difficult. Both local muscle and regional fasciocutaneous flaps have been described with varied levels of success. In this article, the authors describe their case series of 3 patients with long-term osteomyelitis. The interesting thing

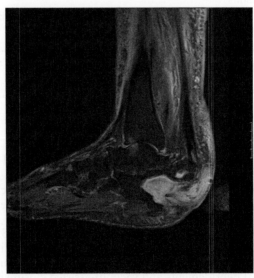

FIGURE 7.—Postoperative MRI showing good flap perfusion. (Reprinted from Ghods M, Grabs R, Kersten C, et al. A modified free muscle transfer technique to effectively treat chronic and persistent calcaneal osteomyelitis. *Ann Plast Surg.* 2012;68:599-605, with permission from Lippincott Williams & Wilkins.)

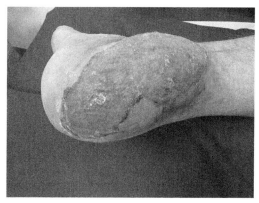

FIGURE 8.—The flap healed uneventfully. (Reprinted from Ghods M, Grabs R, Kersten C, et al. A modified free muscle transfer technique to effectively treat chronic and persistent calcaneal osteomyelitis. *Ann Plast Surg.* 2012;68:599-605, with permission from Lippincott Williams & Wilkins.)

they do (which some other authors have described too) is to radically debride the cancellous bone but leave as much of the cortical bone as possible. After debridement, they interpose a free gracilis flap into the cavity (Figs 7 and 8) and keep the patient nonweight bearing until the flap heals, with the goal of full weight bearing at 2 months. An obvious concern is replacing cancellous bone with muscle and wondering how strong the remaining calcaneus could be and whether it is at risk for refracture. One of their referenced papers describes taking the patient back to the operating room 3 months after gracilis interposition and placing a bone graft to support the calcaneus. It will be interesting to see if bone grafting is truly necessary or could be done selectively on patients who might later require it.

J. Boehmler, MD

Foot and Ankle Reconstruction: Pedicled Muscle Flaps versus Free Flaps and the Role of Diabetes
Ducic I, Attinger CE (Georgetown Univ Hosp, Washington, DC)
Plast Reconstr Surg 128:173-180, 2011

Background.—The effectiveness of pedicled muscle flaps versus microsurgical free flaps in patients with diabetes mellitus for complex foot and ankle reconstruction has not been well defined.

Methods.—The Georgetown Wound Registry identified all patients who underwent pedicled muscle flap or free flap reconstruction from 1990 to 2000 with 8.1 ± 3.1-year follow-up. Thirty-eight diabetic and 42 nondiabetic patients were identified. Flap coverage was the reconstructive choice for defects with exposed tendons, joints, or bone, with pedicled muscle flaps always selected for smaller defects.

Results.—Thirty-two patients received 34 pedicled muscle flaps for 34 wounds, whereas 48 received 52 free flaps for 51 wounds. Thirty-one of

34 wounds covered with pedicled muscle flaps went on to heal, for a 91 percent success rate, a 94 percent limb salvage rate, and a 78 percent patient survival rate. There were 15 complications among 45 reconstructive procedures, for an overall 33 percent complication rate. Forty-eight of the 51 wounds covered with free flaps went on to heal, for a 94 percent healing rate, a 96 percent limb salvage rate, and a 77 percent patient survival rate. There were 17 complications among 93 reconstructive procedures, for an 18 percent complication rate.

Conclusions.—Diabetes does not appear to affect the success of pedicled muscle flap or free flap reconstruction except for requiring more débridements, longer healing times, and decreased long-term survival. When compared with historical diabetic controls with amputation, however, limb salvage appears to prolong survival of diabetic patients. Pedicled muscle flaps appear to be as effective as free flaps for the coverage of small complex foot and ankle defects, despite the postoperative complication rate. Diabetes is not a contraindication to either type of flap reconstruction for limb salvage.

Clinical Question/Level of Evidence.—Therapeutic, III.

▶ This article presents information particularly useful in the management of foot and ankle wounds in diabetic patients. Although some may assume that the transfer of free tissue for coverage of such wounds will result in improved wound healing and more reliable limb salvage because of "better blood supply" than local flaps, this study refutes that assumption. Local flaps, particularly local muscle flaps, provided perfectly effective coverage in appropriate cases. Thus the decision for the surgeon who is considering the use of a local flap or who is perhaps not particularly comfortable with free-flap reconstruction, comes down to the size of the defect. A small defect that can be covered with local muscle does not need a free flap for limb salvage, even in the diabetic patient. Only the defects too large for available local flaps require the use of free tissue transfer. The authors also emphasize that the entire defect does not have to be covered by muscle as long as debridement of all tissues is adequate and exposed bone and tendon are covered by the muscle. Finally, it is especially encouraging to learn from this study that not only can limbs be salvaged using this approach, but these patients actually survive longer if their limbs are preserved.

R. L. Ruberg, MD

Management of Regional Hidradenitis Suppurativa With Vacuum-Assisted Closure and Split Thickness Skin Grafts
Chen E, Friedman HI (Univ of South Carolina School of Medicine, Columbia)
Ann Plast Surg 67:397-401, 2011

Background.—Hidradenitis suppurativa can be a debilitating chronic illness. The underlying cause of the disease is still not clear, but effective treatment of widespread regional disease relies on resection of all the involved skin and subcutaneous tissue. Closure of the resulting large wound is dependent on either flap or skin graft coverage. Many of the resulting wounds are too large for flap closure or result in unacceptable flap donor site deficits.

Methods.—We present a series of 11 patients with 24 regional disease sites treated with a protocol of excision, followed by wound vacuum-assisted closure (VAC; KCI, San Antonio, TX) therapy to stimulate angiogenesis of exposed fat, and then skin grafting with the use of VAC to support the grafts on the recipient sites.

Results.—Only 3 of the patients required regrafting. One patient had a VAC failure because of poor patient compliance, and 1 patient had 4 sites that each required regrafting as the epithelium would not fill in the residual open areas as it usually did in other patients. All patients were cured of their local disease.

Conclusions.—Massive regional hidradenitis suppurativa can be successfully managed with wide excision, VAC therapy, and skin grafting to allow these patients to live normal and productive lives.

▶ Successful treatment of severe hidradenitis suppurativa (HA) can be a vexing problem for even the most skilled plastic surgeon. I applaud the authors for the use of vacuum-assisted drainage to prepare the wounds created after excision of HA and am surprised that more reports of the use of this technique have not appeared in the literature. The suggestion to use stoma adhesive to secure the wound vacuum-assisted closure (VAC) device in the perineal and groin areas is a good suggestion. It would be of great interest to study the comparative results of VAC-assisted wound closure and skin graft with complete excision of affected tissues down to healthy muscle and skin graft regarding success rates as well as the respective costs incurred with each.

S. H. Miller, MD

3 Trauma

Head and Neck

Open reduction versus endoscopically controlled reconstruction of orbital floor fractures: a retrospective analysis

Hundepool AC, Willemsen MAP, Koudstaal MJ, et al (Erasmus Univ Med Ctr, Rotterdam, The Netherlands)
Int J Oral Maxillofac Surg 41:489-493, 2012

The aim of this study was to compare the postoperative results of open reduction versus endoscopically controlled reconstructions of orbital floor fractures. The medical records of 83 patients, treated between January 2000 and December 2008, were reviewed for enophthalmos, diplopia and complications. Fifty-eight patients were operated on using open reduction and in 25 patients the open reduction was endoscopically controlled. A significantly better outcome, regarding enophthalmos and diplopia improvement, was found in the endoscopically controlled

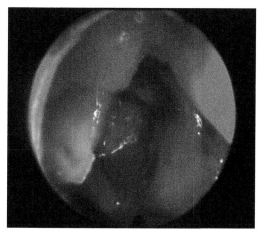

FIGURE 2.—Endoscopic view of the orbital floor from the maxillary sinus before repair. (Reprinted from Hundepool AC, Willemsen MAP, Koudstaal MJ, et al. Open reduction versus endoscopically controlled reconstruction of orbital floor fractures: a retrospective analysis. *Int J Oral Maxillofac Surg.* 2012;41:489-493, with permission from International Association of Oral and Maxillofacial Surgeons.)

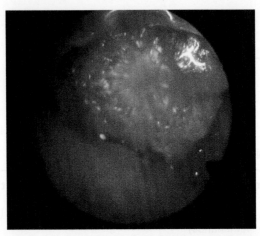

FIGURE 3.—Endoscopic view of orbital floor from the maxillary sinus after repair. (Reprinted from Hundepool AC, Willemsen MAP, Koudstaal MJ, et al. Open reduction versus endoscopically controlled reconstruction of orbital floor fractures: a retrospective analysis. *Int J Oral Maxillofac Surg.* 2012;41:489-493, Copyright 2012, with permission from International Association of Oral and Maxillofacial Surgeons.)

group. Endoscopically controlled reconstruction of orbital floor fractures seems to be a more accurate and successful treatment (Figs 2 and 3).

▶ This is a very large retrospective series from the Netherlands documenting the results of treating orbital floor fractures by an open technique (group 1) versus open technique plus endoscopic-controlled reconstruction (group 2).[1] Questions arise as to the reason the authors chose to report the results for 83 patients of the original 171 treated by them without a specific explanation. Although the retrospective analysis seems to indicate no real differences in a variety of variables between the 2 groups other than the most common etiology in group 1 was "violence" and in group 2 it was "traffic accidents," the 2 groups were treated at different time intervals. The results clearly establish, in this study, the benefits of using the endoscopic-aided approach regarding both enophthalmos and improvement in the level of postreduction diplopia, but would have been more convincing if the 2 groups had been randomized a priori (Figs 2 and 3). Another question to be addressed is whether the use of harvested bone grafts for repair of the floor is a better option than the use of other biological and nonbiological materials.[2]

S. H. Miller, MD

References

1. Saunders CJ, Whetzel TP, Stokes RB, Wong GB, Stevenson TR. Transantral endoscopic orbital floor exploration: a cadaver and clinical study. *Plast Reconstr Surg.* 1997;100:575-581.
2. Persons BL, Wong GB. Transantral endoscopic orbital floor repair using resorbable plate. *J Crainofac Surg.* 2002;113:483-488.

Lip replantation: A viable option for lower lip reconstruction after human bites, a literature review and proposed management algorithm
Liliav B, Zaluzec R, Hassid VJ, et al (Univ of Illinois at Chicago)
J Plast Reconstr Aesthet Surg 65:e197-e199, 2012

Background.—Rarely do cases of traumatic lip amputation by human bite occur. As a result, there is no universally accepted protocol for managing lip amputations from human bites. A case treated with lip replantation was reported.

    Case Report.—Man, 64, was assessed for about 50% lip amputation after a human bite. The severely contused amputated lip had been wrapped in saline-soaked gauze and placed on ice. The right labial artery was avulsed and retracted. Surgery was performed immediately, with devitalized and crushed tissues debrided and the right and left labial arteries anastomosed to their original sources. No veins were available for anastomosis. After reconstruction the replanted lip was pink and viable. Leech therapy was used for 8 days combined with prophylactic subcutaneous heparin and aspirin. Ten days after surgery the inferior border of the replanted lip demonstrated epidermolysis, requiring the operative debridement of nonviable tissue. The final result was satisfactory functionally and esthetically.

Conclusions.—Successful lip replantation requires rapid clinical assessment and management using adequate microsurgical skills. Cases usually require anticoagulation; low-dose dextran, intra-replant heparin, subcutaneous heparin, and aspirin can be used for this. Leech therapy and pin prick technique may also be used. Replantation also involves at least end-to-end anastomosis of the right and left inferior labial artery. Possible complications include venous congestion, partial tissue loss, continued bleeding from suture sites, and acute blood loss. Red blood cell transfusion can also be needed.

▶ Faced with a similar type of injury in a young patient, a 15-year-old male, involving avulsion of approximately one third of the upper lip plus a significant portion of the lower half of the nose, we replanted the tissue and anastomosed the two labial arteries, but could find no suitable veins. We then proceeded to treat the patient with daily aspirin and leeches for 8 days. Fortunately, virtually all of the tissue survived. Despite initial concerns that the leaches might enter his nose or mouth, the patient bore up well and was quite pleased that his injury was immediately repaired in one step and achieved a good aesthetic result. The algorithm proposed by the authors is a commonsense approach to these unusual problems, not just for human bites, but for animal bites and other causes of lip and nose avulsion injuries as well.

S. H. Miller, MD

Extremity and Trunk

Early soft tissue coverage and negative pressure wound therapy optimises patient outcomes in lower limb trauma

Liu DSH, Sofiadellis F, Ashton M, et al (The Royal Melbourne Hosp, Parkville, Victoria, Australia)
Injury 43:772-778, 2012

Background.—The timing of soft tissue reconstruction for severe open lower limb trauma is critical to its successful outcome, particularly in the setting of exposed metalware and pre-existing wound infection. The use of negative pressure wound therapy (NPWT) may allow a delay in soft tissue coverage without adverse effects. This study evaluated the impact of delayed free-flap reconstruction, prolonged metalware exposure, pre-flap wound infection, and the efficacy of NPWT on the success of soft tissue coverage after open lower limb injury.

Methods.—Retrospective review of all free-flap reconstructions for lower limb trauma undertaken at a tertiary trauma centre between June 2002 and July 2009.

Results.—103 patients underwent 105 free-flap reconstructions. Compared with patients who were reconstructed within 3 days of injury, the cohort with delayed reconstruction beyond 7 days had significantly increased rates of pre-flap wound infection, flap re-operation, deep metal infection and osteomyelitis. Pre-flap wound infection independently predicted adverse surgical outcomes. In the setting of exposed metalware, free-flap transfer beyond one day significantly increased the flap failure rate. These patients required more surgical procedures and a longer hospital stay. The use of NPWT significantly lowered the rate of flap re-operations and venous thrombosis, but did not allow a delay in reconstruction beyond 7 days from injury without a concomitant rise in skeletal and flap complications.

Conclusions.—Following open lower limb trauma, soft tissue coverage within 3 days of injury and immediately following fracture fixation with exposed metalware minimises pre-flap wound infection and optimises surgical outcomes. NPWT provides effective temporary wound coverage, but does not allow a delay in definitive free-flap reconstruction.

▶ As they say—what's old is new again. In the early days of microsurgery, Marco Godina published an authoritative article on the outcomes of early microsurgical intervention for lower extremity trauma. In his landmark study of his experience of more than 500 cases, he found a significant improvement in the flap survival, limb salvage rates, bone healing rates, and hospitalization days for patients who underwent flap coverage within 72 hours of their injury. Since then, negative pressure wound therapy (NPWT) has become a commonly utilized wound dressing, and some have advocated that NPWT can decrease the need for microsurgery and complications. However, in this well-executed (and statistically heavy) study, the authors found that for patients who required free-flap reconstruction, the same rule of flap coverage within 72 hours applies for optimal outcomes. In addition, they found that orthopedic hardware that was exposed in the wound for more than 1 day had increased rates of complications. They summarized that although the NPWT can provide a good temporary coverage, it is not the magic elixir to allow for delayed flap reconstruction. Unfortunately, it would have been interesting to see how many of their trauma patients were able to avoid free-flap reconstruction because of NPWT, but those data were not presented. A good take-home message from this study is that if a free flap is likely needed for a lower extremity trauma case, it's best not to delay but rather to get it done as soon as possible, especially if metallic hardware is exposed. Any plastic surgeon who cares for lower extremity patients would be wise to review this article.

J. Boehmler, MD

Outcomes of anterolateral thigh free flap thinning using liposuction following lower limb trauma

Askouni EP, Topping A, Ball S, et al (Imperial College Healthcare NHS Trust, London, UK)
J Plast Reconstr Aesthet Surg 65:474-481, 2012

Background.—Whilst soft tissue closure is the priority to prevent infection in open fractures of the lower limb, some patients find that bulky flaps interfere with function and dislike the appearance. We report the outcomes of delayed free anterolateral thigh flap thinning with liposuction.

Material and Methods.—38 patients treated between 2006 and 2009 were offered flap contouring. 23 chose flap thinning and 15 did not. We measured outcomes using the SF-36v2 questionnaire and cosmetic outcome scores pre and postoperatively at a mean follow up of 12 weeks (range 10—16 weeks).

Results.—SF-36v2 physical health (PH) scores improved from a mean of 67 preoperatively to 80 postoperatively ($p = 0.01$) in the thinned group, while mental health (MH) scores remained unchanged (74—72). The mean SF-36v2 scores for the non-thinned group were 77 (PH) and 86 (MH). Following liposuction the median cosmetic outcome scores out of 5 improved from 1 (not at all satisfied) to 4 (very satisfied) postoperatively ($p = 0.0005$), which was also higher than the non-thinned group (3) [moderately satisfied], $p = 0.004$. There was no difference in sex, age, BMI and region on the leg of free flap reconstruction between the non-thinned and thinned groups.

Conclusions.—Delayed contouring of free ALT flaps used for lower limb reconstruction results in improvements in physical health measures and cosmetic outcomes. Patients not requesting thinning are generally satisfied with their reconstruction (Fig 2).

▶ There continues to be significant controversy regarding the role of fasciocutaneous versus muscle flaps in reconstructing distal extremities. The group in favor

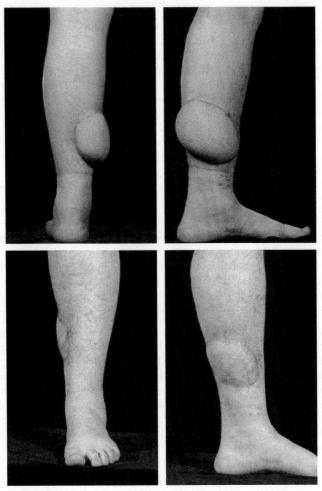

FIGURE 2.—ALT flap used to cover a middle third tibial fracture in a 32 year old male patient. Figures demonstrate appearance pre-thinning (top left and right) and post-thinning (bottom left and right). (Reprinted from Askouni EP, Topping A, Ball S, et al. Outcomes of anterolateral thigh free flap thinning using liposuction following lower limb trauma. *J Plast Reconstr Aesthet Surg.* 2012;65:474-481, with permission from British Association of Plastic, Reconstructive and Aesthetic Surgeons.)

of muscle flaps remarks on the good aesthetics of the reconstruction, especially when a sheet skin graft is used. Although it will take time for the muscle to atrophy, the flap frequently will contour well. This article from the United Kingdom adequately shows that better cosmetic outcomes can be obtained with liposuction and revising fasciocutaneous flaps (in this case the anterolateral thigh [ALT] flap), but I wonder how the cosmetic outcome would have compared to a series of muscle flap reconstructions. Fig 2 presents a case that seems to have been a great opportunity for a serratus flap with skin graft. With the ALT flap, there is a high likelihood of needing a revision, where it is much less likely after a muscle flap, which is not addressed in this article. It would have been helpful for them to mention how the liposuction and revision is reimbursed (insurance? self-pay?), as some payors may consider this cosmetic. Although the debate will continue which flap to continue, this group is to be congratulated on the aesthetic reconstruction they are able to eventually achieve.

J. Boehmler, MD

Burns

"The Maestro": A Pioneering Plastic Surgeon—Sir Archibald McIndoe and His Innovating Work on patients With Burn Injury During World War II
Geomelas M, Ghods M, Ring A, et al (Ernst von Bergmann Hosp, Potsdam, Germany; Ruhr-Univ Bochum, Berlin, Germany; et al)
J Burn Care Res 32:363-368, 2011

This article describes McIndoe's revolutionary methods of burn treatment and rehabilitation of patients with burn injury and outlines his personality traits that made him one of the most important plastic surgeons of the twentieth century. As a consultant plastic surgeon to the Royal Air Force, he set up a plastic surgery unit in the Queen Victoria Hospital in East Grinstead. By using biographical data and photography, McIndoe's work on burns treatment and the challenges he faced are presented. Before World War II, little was known about the treatment of severe burns and their complications, and even less was done about the rehabilitation and social reintegration of patients with burn injury. McIndoe changed all that by developing new techniques for the management and reconstruction of burn injuries. He helped his patients become and get accepted as a normal part of society again. The patients with burn injury treated by him formed the Guinea Pig Club. Sir Archibald Hector McIndoe, a charismatic plastic surgeon with an uncanny instinctive knowledge of psychology, recognized early that the rehabilitation of a burned patient was as important as the reconstruction of his physical body. His therapeutic approach to patients with burn injury was mental and physical.

▶ This is a must read. Sadly, many young trainees in plastic surgery do not know or care about the giants who preceded them. McIndoe was a hero and worthy of emulation. The history of our profession is fascinating and should be required reading.

R. Salisbury, MD

The Elimination of Postburn Nasal Contracture in Children With Trapeze-Flap Plasty

Grishkevich VM (A.V. Vishnevsky Inst of Surgery of the Russian Academy of Med Sciences, Moscow, Russia)
J Burn Care Res 32:566-569, 2011

One consequence of a facial burn is nasal contracture. In pediatric patients, scar tension presents a particular problem because of facial growth. The forehead and nasal scar contraction deform the nose dorsum, especially between the eyes. The nasofrontal angle becomes smoothened, wide, and flat; the scar edges cover the inner canthus. The dorsum nose scar stretching delays nasal development, pulls the nose up, making it shorter, and causes nasal ectropion. Secondary deformity of the nose's solid structures develops as a consequence of scar contracture, and its reconstruction poses a major problem. At the same time, it is suggested that nasal reconstruction in the pediatric patients should be planned as a staged procedure. Therefore, scar contracture release should be performed early, at the first stage of pediatric nasal reconstruction, to create conditions for normal nasal development. In this author's opinion, the most suitable procedure is trapeze-flap plasty. The scar tissue surplus in the nasofrontal angle allows contracture release with local tissues. Reconstruction with local trapezoid flaps releases the scar tension and elongates the nasal dorsum surface by approximately 1.5 cm; the epicanthus is eliminated, and the nasofrontal angle (nasal root) is restored. Eight children were operated. Good results were observed in all patients for the duration of 3 years.

▶ I commend the author on addressing this very challenging and problematic deformity, particularly as it complicates the course and recovery of the pediatric burn survivor. The use of local flaps remains one of the most valuable tools in the armamentarium of the burn and reconstructive surgeon, and thankfully there is significant precedent establishing the successful use of burned tissue in the design of local flaps.

The author has described the application of a flap design that works well in his hands for the release of multiple burn contracture deformities, and while similar to opposing Z-plasties, its geometric design differs and may prove beneficial when a narrowed concentric result is desirable.

Total nasal reconstruction, using forehead flaps, cartilaginous grafts, prefabricated and free microvascular transfers, as well as a variety of full dorsal resurfacing techniques, has an established role in complex nasal deformities and yet, not every patient is a good candidate for these reconstructive procedures (some might prefer less involved reconstructive options). It is here that techniques such as those described in this article may be a worthwhile option. The end result may prove quite satisfactory both aesthetically and functionally, and, perhaps as important, future reconstructive options are not compromised. The release of local tension over time has proven beneficial in scar remodeling, so there is a sound basis for its use in the pediatric patient.

It would be interesting to have long-term follow-up in order to evaluate the skeletal, developmental, and functional end results.

M. Tennenhaus, MD

Medial sural perforator plus island flap: A modification of the medial sural perforator island flap for the reconstruction of postburn knee flexion contractures using burned calf skin
Kim KS, Kim ES, Hwang JH, et al (Chonnam Natl Univ Med School, Dong-gu, Gwangju, Korea)
J Plast Reconstr Aesthet Surg 65:804-809, 2012

Background.—The medial sural perforator island flap may be suitable for the reconstruction of postburn knee flexion contractures. However, postburn knee flexion contractures are usually associated with burns of the calf, which is the donor site of the medial sural perforator flap. Thus, there are concerns regarding the safety of raising medial sural perforator flaps from burned calves.

Methods.—Between 2005 and 2010, 12 patients (11 males and 1 female) with postburn knee flexion contractures associated with second-degree burns of the calf (that healed by secondary intention) underwent reconstruction using a medial sural perforator island flap (based on the medial sural perforator) or medial sural perforator plus island flap (based on the medial sural perforator and other vessels that are pedicles of the sural flaps).

Results.—All 12 flaps, which ranged in size from 7 to 15 cm in width and from 9 to 23 cm in length, survived completely. Of the 12 flaps, three were medial sural perforator island flaps and nine were medial sural perforator plus island flaps. Of the nine medial sural perforator plus island flaps, two included the lesser saphenous vein, five included the lesser saphenous vein and its accompanying artery, and two included the lesser saphenous vein, the distal sural nerve and their accompanying arteries. Healing of all donor sites was uncomplicated. All patients were completely satisfied with their results.

Conclusions.—Although this series is not large, the authors are convinced that some reliable medial sural perforators are usually present under second-degree burned calf skin that healed by secondary intention, and that the medial sural perforator island flap or the medial sural perforator plus island flap can be safely used even though the skin may not be as pliable as normal skin (Fig 4).

▶ This surgery is not meant for the weak-willed or faint of heart. The medial sural artery perforator flap is a wonderful flap that is not utilized in the United States nearly enough but has the potential of being a nice alternative to the radial forearm or the anterolateral thigh flap. It has a relatively long pedicle and can take a fairly large, thin, and pliable skin paddle. In cases of anterior knee coverage, it can be a nice (and less morbid) alternative to the gastrocnemius if a muscle flap is not necessarily needed. In this article, the authors up the ante in the treatment of burn

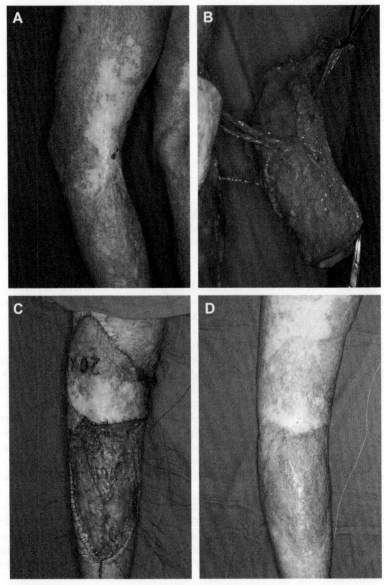

FIGURE 4.—A 65-year-old man with flexion contracture around the left popliteal area (patient 11 in Table 1). (A) Preoperative view. (B) Flap elevation. After the contracture had been completely released, a 15 × 20-cm medial sural perforator plus island flap, based on 3 medial sural perforators, the lesser saphenous vein and sural nerve, their accompanying arteries and another superficial vein, was raised. (C) Immediate postoperative view. The raised flap was transposed and sutured to the defect, and the flap donor site was covered with a split-thickness skin graft. (D) Long-term follow-up view. The patient demonstrated a full range of knee motion and functional and cosmetic results were satisfactory at 15 months postoperatively. (Reprinted from Kim KS, Kim ES, Hwang JH, et al. Medial sural perforator plus island flap: a modification of the medial sural perforator island flap for the reconstruction of postburn knee flexion contractures using burned calf skin. *J Plast Reconstr Aesthet Surg.* 2012;65:804-809, Copyright 2012, with permission from British Association of Plastic, Reconstructive and Aesthetic Surgeons.)

patients with anterior knee contractures by not only utilizing this flap for coverage, but by using a flap that was involved in the burn to begin with. All 12 patients had second-degree burns of the medial calf but, after allowing for secondary healing, found they were able to successfully transfer these flaps without complication. This does make sense considering that the donor sites were only affected with partial thickness burns, and the deep structures like blood supply should be preserved. In the majority of the cases (9 of 12), they brought a secondary blood supply with the flap, creating the medial sural perforator plus flap, usually the lesser saphenous vein (Fig 4). This additional venous outflow is likely beneficial because the flaps were frequently stiffer from their secondary healing and were not as pliable as nonburned tissue. Although they used handheld Doppler for their preoperative perforator analysis, this might be a good indication for indocyanine green fluorescence to evaluate for perforator and skin perfusion. Hopefully, with this article, and others like it, the medial sural artery perforator flap will become more commonly utilized, especially around the knee, as it allows for a large flap reconstruction without requiring microsurgery.

J. Boehmler, MD

Virtual reality for acute pain reduction in adolescents undergoing burn wound care: A prospective randomized controlled trial
Kipping B, Rodger S, Miller K, et al (Queensland Children's Med Res Inst, Brisbane, Australia; The Univ of Queensland, Brisbane, Australia)
Burns 38:650-657, 2012

Background.—Effective pain management remains a challenge for adolescents during conscious burn wound care procedures. Virtual reality (VR) shows promise as a non-pharmacological adjunct in reducing pain.

Aims.—This study assessed off-the-shelf VR for (1) its effect on reducing acute pain intensity during adolescent burn wound care, and (2) its clinical utility in a busy hospital setting.

Methods.—Forty-one adolescents (11–17 years) participated in this prospective randomized controlled trial. Acute pain outcomes including adolescent self-report, nursing staff behavioral observation, caregiver observation and physiological measures were collected. Length of procedure times and adolescent reactions were also recorded to inform clinical utility.

Results.—Nursing staff reported a statistically significant reduction in pain scores during dressing removal, and significantly less rescue doses of Entonox given to those receiving VR, compared to those receiving standard distraction. For all other pain outcomes and length of treatment, there was a trend for lower pain scores and treatment times for those receiving VR, but these differences were not statistically significant.

Conclusion.—Despite only minimal pain reduction achieved using off-the-shelf VR, other results from this trial and previous research on younger

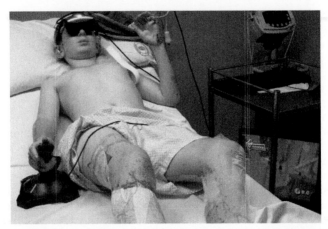

FIGURE 1.—Picture of an adolescent using the off-the-shelf VR system. (Reprinted from Kipping B, Rodger S, Miller K, et al. Virtual reality for acute pain reduction in adolescents undergoing burn wound care: a prospective randomized controlled trial. *Burns*. 2012;38:650-657, Copyright 2012, with permission from International Society for Burn Injuries.)

children with burns suggest a customized, adolescent and hospital friendly device may be more effective in pain reduction (Fig 1).

▶ If you ever need to trim a large dog's toenails, a great trick is to give it a nearly empty jar of peanut butter. While he is rummaging in there for the last little bit, you're free to do just about anything you want to him, and it makes nail trimming a much less painful ordeal (for both you and your companion). This is known as the *Gate Control* theory of pain, when the brain is distracted from a painful stimulus. Unfortunately, adolescent burn patients are not as easily distracted with peanut butter as greyhounds are, so more imaginative methods need to be applied to assist with their care, particularly during dressing changes. In this study, the authors compared a virtual reality (VR) system that allowed the patient to play an age-appropriate game (Fig 1) to standard distraction techniques of music, TV, and stories. The only outcomes that were significantly in favor of the VR distraction system were the number of rescue pain medications administered and the pain intensity at dressing removal as measured by the nurses (but not the patients). Unfortunately, this study was likely limited by a lack of statistical power, as there were some trends that were there in favor of VR but did not achieve significance. They also mentioned that this VR system was an off-the-shelf option and described more expensive, customizable, VR systems that might have more of an effect. Personally, I think the major limitation of this experience presented was that the kids had only a small selection of games to play. Given how many kids play video games these days, it would seem reasonable to allow them to play whatever XBox, Playstation, or Wii game they wanted. These game consoles are going to be cheaper than any VR system, and, if visual isolation is required like they have for the VR system, monitor eyeglasses are coming into the marketplace that could fit the bill. Because most pediatric units have video game consoles available, it would be relatively easy to perform a similar study and include all patients who undergo dressing changes for any reason (eg, burn, trauma, infection) to get better numbers. Discovering ways to decrease the pain and trauma of dressing changes to kids without the use of narcotics can only be seen as a worthy endeavor, and I applaud the authors for their early work on this topic.

J. Boehmler, MD

Use of split thickness plantar skin grafts in the treatment of hyperpigmented skin-grafted fingers and palms in previously burned patients

Moon S-H, Lee S-Y, Jung S-N, et al (Catholic Univ of Korea, Uijongbu)
Burns 37:714-720, 2011

Palmar and finger burns are often seen in children, and are usually as a result of contact burns. Some patients with deep hand burns are treated with full-thickness or split-thickness skin grafts. Skin graft is commonly used for hand reconstruction. However, the grafted skin would be more pigmented than the adjacent skin and different from skin texture.

19 patients who showed hyperpigmentation after skin graft of finger and palm were treated. They all were injured by hand burns. We performed mechanical dermabrasion of the hyperpigmentation scar and application of a split thickness skin harvested from medial aspect of plantar of foot. Patients were asked about their level of satisfaction with the procedure and scar appearance was assessed using a five-point Likert scale. Also scar appearances were assessed using a Vancouver Scar Scale (VSS).

The grafts were completely taken in all 19 patients. The color of the graft became similar to adjacent tissue. 15 patients were very satisfied, and four patients were relatively satisfied. The average score of the patients postoperative appearance improvement was 4.5 (improved to significantly improved postoperative appearance). Average VSS score was improved from 9.53 to 2.53. There was no hypertrophic scar on plantar donor site.

The technique of the split-thickness plantar skin graft after mechanical dermabrasion is simple and provided good results in both color and texture for the patients who showed hyperpigmentation after grafting (Fig 3).

▶ Plantar and palmar non-hair-bearing skin are quite similar to one another, and use of the former, as a split-thickness graft, to replace pigmented skin grafts on the hands of children following burns, is a rational approach to improve cosmesis.[1] Caveats to consider are the down time caused by pain and healing at the donor site as well as the need for careful placement of the new grafts to minimize potential functional loss. One of my concerns was that the pre- and postoperative photographs were not taken using the same background and lighting. This oversight make judging the cosmetic result somewhat problematic (Fig 3).

S. H. Miller, MD

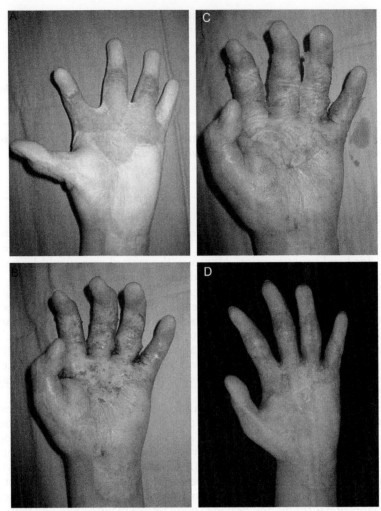

FIGURE 3.—15 year-old male who had been injured by contact burn 14 years ago was treated with mechanical dermabrasion and plantar STSG. (A) Preoperative view, (B) intra-operative view, post-dermabrasion, (C) raw surface covered with STSG, (D) one year after operation. (Reprinted from Moon S-H, Lee S-Y, Jung S-N, et al. Use of split thickness plantar skin grafts in the treatment of hyper-pigmented skin-grafted fingers and palms in previously burned patients. *Burns.* 2011;37:714-720, Copyright 2011, with permission from International Society for Burn Injuries.)

Reference

1. Roboti EB, Edstrom LE. Split-thickness plantar grafts for coverage in the hands and digits. *J Hand Surg Am.* 1991;16:143-146.

A Case Report of Doxycycline-Induced Stevens–Johnson Syndrome

Lau B, Mutyala D, Dhaliwal D (Univ of Pittsburgh Med School, PA; Univ of Pittsburgh Med Ctr, PA)
Cornea 30:595-597, 2011

Purpose.—To report the clinical findings of a case of Stevens–Johnson syndrome (SJS) precipitated by the use of systemic doxycycline.

Methods.—Case report.

Results.—A 49-year-old man developed SJS with ocular involvement after doxycycline use for respiratory symptoms. The patient developed persistent 2+ conjunctival injection and foreshortening of the conjunctival fornices in both eyes. The right eye had a 3 × 3.4 mm corneal epithelial defect with 50% thinning. The left eye had a 2.6 × 3 mm corneal ulcer with a central perforation and a flat anterior chamber with 360 degrees of iridocorneal touch.

Conclusions.—This case illustrates the unusual presentation of SJS induced by doxycycline. The prevalent use of systemic doxycycline in the practice of ophthalmology for eyelid-related and ocular surface disorders coupled with the detrimental long-term sequelae of SJS renders a careful reevaluation for alternatives.

▶ This case report is interesting because it confirms that any antibiotic can cause defoliating disease. This patient did not have Stevens-Johnson syndrome, but the more virulent toxic epidermal necrolysis (TEN). While part of the same spectrum, TEN involves greater than 30% of the body surface, which was the case in this patient. The prognosis is much worse and the complications more frequent.

R. Salisbury, MD

4 Hand and Upper Extremity

Surgical Hand Antisepsis for the Hand Surgeon

Katz DI, Watson JT (Vanderbilt Orthopaedic Inst, Nashville, TN)
J Hand Surg 36A:1706-1707, 2011

Background.—Surgical hand antisepsis removes transient microorganisms and reduces the number of resident microorganisms on the surgeon's hands. It is designed to lower the risk of surgical site infection (SSI), which is the most common nosocomial infection among surgical patients. Because sterile gloves can become perforated, it is desirable to keep the hands as germfree as possible. The most commonly used methods to achieve surgical hand antisepsis were described and compared.

Methods.—Attributes of an ideal antiseptic agent are fast action, persistence, cumulative action, broad-spectrum activity, and safety. The three types of solutions used are aqueous scrubs, alcohol rubs, and alcohol rubs with added active ingredients. The most common aqueous scrub agents are povidone iodine (PI) and chlorhexidine gluconate (CHG). Ethanol, isopropanol, and n-propanol are the typical alcohol rubs, which are 60% to 90% in strength. The most common active ingredients added to alcohol rubs are biguanides (chlorhexidine) and phenolic compounds (triclosan). These combine alcohol's rapid bacteriocidal effects with aqueous scrubs' persistent chemical activity. PI and CHG are usually used preoperatively as surgical hand scrubs. Although PI acts immediately and covers a broad spectrum of bacteria, it has little to no residual effect on colonizing bacteria. CHG adds to the immediate and broad-spectrum activity the ability to bind to the skin's outermost layer (the stratum corneum), providing sustained release. Used repeatedly, CHG's effects are cumulative.

Comparisons.—Several studies find CHG is more effective than PI for reducing bacterial colony-forming units (CFUs). CHG also causes substantial and sustained reductions in hand bacterial counts and is better than PI for orthopedic procedures. Alcohol-based rubs used in orthopedic procedures had rates of SSIs equivalent to those of PI and CHG. In addition, alcohol-based rubs cause less skin irritation and dryness and improve compliance with use. Comparing an alcohol-based waterless rub, an alcohol-based water-aided scrub solution, and a traditional PI aqueous scrub showed no difference in CFU reductions between the three, but the alcohol-based waterless rub was less irritating and was preferred by participants.

Conclusions.—The main conclusions regarding surgical hand antisepsis are (1) that CHG scrubs are more effective than PI scrubs for reducing the number of CFUs on hands and (2) that alcohol-based rubs are at least as effective or more effective than traditional aqueous scrubs. The frequent use of aqueous antiseptics and traumatic scrubbing techniques produces skin irritation and allergic reactions. Alcohol rubs require less time to apply and can improve compliance among surgical team members. Alcohol agents may also be cheaper than traditional scrubs with brushes. Further studies are needed.

▶ This is not a topic we spend a lot of time discussing. This article is a short, concise, clear review of current available hand washing techniques. The debunking of nail cleaning or a traditional scrub as the first of the day is refreshing. Cost and time are mentioned but not quantitated. This will be more important in the future.

D. J. Smith, Jr, MD

Rice Bodies, Millet Seeds, and Melon Seeds in Tuberculous Tenosynovitis of the Hand and Wrist
Woon CY-L, Phoon E-S, Lee JY-L, et al (Singapore General Hosp; Natl Univ Hosp, Singapore)
Ann Plast Surg 66:610-617, 2011

Tuberculosis (TB) is still endemic in many developed countries. Involvement of the hand and wrist at presentation is extremely rare, and the diagnosis is often missed. Operative findings of "rice bodies, millet seeds, or melon seeds" are highly suggestive of tuberculous tenosynovitis. Six patients with TB of the hand and wrist at various stages of disease with characteristic operative findings are reviewed. Four patients had underlying immunosuppression. One patient had previous pulmonary TB, whereas 3 patients had radiographic evidence of previously undiagnosed pulmonary TB. The interval to presentation ranged from 1 week to 2 years. Two patients had median nerve irritation, 3 patients had osteomyelitis, and 1 patient had flexor tendon rupture. Mycobacterial cultures were positive in 4 patients; acid-fast bacilli stain, and polymerase chain reaction were positive in remaining 1 patient; and both stain and culture were negative in the last patient who had history of pulmonary TB. All 6 patients were managed with combination therapy comprising antituberculous chemotherapy and at least 1 debulking tenosynovectomy. Two patients had 2 debridements. Of these 2 patients, 1 underwent wrist arthrodesis during the second procedure. Mean follow-up was 4 years. There were no recurrences after the most recent debridement. The diagnosis of TB of the hand and wrist is often missed. The surgeon has to be aware of the significance of loose bodies when performing routine excision of innocuous looking wrist ganglia. Combination therapy comprising thorough excisional debridement and antituberculous chemotherapy will minimize recurrence of this difficult-to-treat disease.

► It has been long time since I've seen a case of tuberculosis (TB) in the hand or wrist. It is well accepted that there is a resurgence of TB, which may increase the likelihood of encountering these patients. Many times, patients will receive medication before seeing the surgeon. Patients may often be seen with a nonspecific tendonitis first. Recently we encountered a tuberculoma of the upper leg. Increased awareness will help patients be treated expeditiously.

D. J. Smith, Jr, MD

Role of Elective Hand Surgery and Tourniquet Use in Patients With Prior Breast Cancer Treatment
Habbu R, Adams JE (Univ of Minnesota, Minneapolis; HealthPartners Inst for Med Education Hand Surgery Fellowship, St Paul, MN)
J Hand Surg 36A:1537-1539, 2011

Background.—When the lymphatic system fails to drain the lymph volume, fluid accumulates in the tissues, producing lymphedema. Breast cancer treatment can affect the lymph system at either the axillary lymph node level or the tissue level. Lymphedema complicates breast cancer treatment in 6% to 70% of cases and is particularly associated with mastectomy, axillary dissection, and irradiation. Because of this association, clinicians often caution patients about or advise them to avoid procedures such as intravenous procedures, injections, blood pressure cuff applications, tourniquet use, or upper limb surgery. Little evidence supports these recommendations. Studies of the occurrence of lymphedema in the affected arm after breast cancer treatment often have problems such as small sample size or the performance of more invasive procedures and treatments that are uncommon today. The guidelines for avoiding lymphedema may need to be reconsidered for elective hand surgery and tourniquet use.

Evidence.—Series investigating elective hand surgery and tourniquet use after breast cancer tend to indicate a low risk of lymphedema. Eight of 15 patients with previous lymph node surgery had no worsening of lymphedema present before surgery and no development of lymphedema not present previously. Thus a history of axillary dissection irradiation may not contraindicate elective hand surgery if routine, proper sterile techniques and surgical measures are used. General anesthesia and short tourniquet use were associated with minimal complications. Pneumatic tourniquets in short procedures had no influence on arm swelling, and history of breast cancer treatment did not affect final outcome. Occasional carpal tunnel decompression may benefit patients with lymphedema. Drawing blood or having an intravenous injection into the arm after breast cancer surgery has a low risk of complications. Routine hand cases were also safe, especially in the absence of lymphedema.

Of 606 hand surgeons polled, about 95% regularly performed elective hand surgery in patients who had previous ipsilateral lymph node excision. Eighty-five percent said they would perform surgery in patients with preexisting lymphedema. Ninety-four percent used a tourniquet in patients who had lymph node dissection and 74% when lymphedema was present. Only 10% felt hand surgery increased the risk of lymphedema; only about 23% believed it would exacerbate any preexisting condition. The Bier block was preferred by 46% of surgeons but only 21% would use it with lymphedema present. Perioperative antibiotics or postoperative therapy was suggested by half of the surgeons. Similarly, 41% of hand surgeons but nearly 80% of breast care team members believed elective hand surgery would be relatively contraindicated if the patient had previous breast cancer treatment. Most hand surgeons would still use a tourniquet.

Summary.—The literature supports performing hand surgery in patients who have undergone breast cancer treatment. It is safe to use regional anesthesia and an upper arm tourniquet. Patients should be told that there is a low risk for lymphedema after hand surgery, especially if their breast cancer treatment included less invasive procedures. Precautions include proper sterile techniques and additional perioperative procedures such as antibiotics, postoperative limb elevation, or postoperative hand therapy. Further study is needed.

▶ This is an excellent review of the role of elective hand surgery and tourniquet in patients with previous breast cancer treatment. There is definitely a paucity of literature on the subject. Any surgeon evaluating these patients should read this review.

D. J. Smith, Jr, MD

Hand Surgery: Considerations in Pregnant Patients
Humbyrd CJ, Laporte DM (The Johns Hopkins Univ, Baltimore, MD)
J Hand Surg 37A:1086-1089, 2012

Background.—Nonobstetric surgical procedures requiring anesthesia are performed in pregnant patients, although elective surgery should be postponed until after delivery. A large meta-analysis on nonobstetric surgery in pregnancy found that maternal mortality is less than 1 in 10,000, it does not raise the risk of major birth defects, and surgery and general anesthesia do not pose major risks for spontaneous abortion. Guidelines for the optimal care of a pregnant patient having hand surgery were offered.

Timing, Monitoring, Anesthesia, and Positioning.—If possible, nonurgent surgery should be done in the second trimester when preterm contractions and spontaneous abortion are less likely. Fetal heart rate should be monitored by Doppler before and after surgery for a previable fetus. Heart rate and contractions should be monitored before, after, and during (when feasible) surgery for a viable fetus. If intraoperative fetal monitoring is used, the patient should give consent for emergency cesarean delivery and the obstetrical team should be readily available.

The physiologic changes of pregnancy nearly all affect anesthesia. Managing the airway is vital, since pregnant patients have 20% greater oxygen consumption and 20% less pulmonary functional residual capacity. Apnea causes a rapid decline in oxygenation. Oropharyngeal swelling and a smaller glottis opening can interfere with intubation and ventilation. Pregnancy reduces lower esophageal sphincter tone, increases gastric acidity, and delays gastric emptying, raising the risk for aspiration pneumonia.

Anesthetic medications tend not to be teratogenic but concerns remain about their ability to cross the placenta and affect the fetus. Regional anesthesia is preferred to general anesthesia where feasible. The lowest placental transfer is seen with spinal anesthesia. There is no restriction on the agents used for local or regional anesthesia. For general anesthesia, neostigmine and atropine are preferred to neostigmine and glycopyrrolate to reverse muscle relaxation.

Uterine displacement to avoid the gravid uterus compressing the inferior vena cava is advised after about 20 to 24 weeks' gestation. The uterus is displaced leftward by 15° to 20° to avoid compression and improve placental flow to the fetus, making the left lateral decubitus position ideal. Other positions are used only with obstetric consultation and intraoperative fetal monitoring.

Perioperative Concerns.—A team consisting of surgical and obstetric personnel should monitor the patient during and after surgery. Thromboembolism risk is increased with pregnancy and more so with surgery, so early mobilization and mechanical prophylaxis with compression stockings and sequential compression devices are advised for all pregnant surgical patients. Chemoprophylaxis is used depending on the length of surgery and thromboembolic risk. Heparin and low-molecular-weight heparin are preferred because they do not cross the placenta. Dextrans run the risk of fetal anaphylaxis leading to fetal distress and should be avoided. Warfarin is a known teratogen that crosses the placenta, so it is also contraindicated in pregnancy. Aspirin and other nonsteroidal anti-inflammatories increase the risk of peripartum hemorrhage, neonatal intracranial hemorrhage, and premature closure of the ductus arteriosus. With respect to antibiotics, only vancomycin raises concern; it should be given only under the guidance and monitoring of the obstetrical team. Other perioperative antibiotics are given on the same dosing schedule and for the same indications as in nonpregnant patients.

Pain increases the risk of premature labor, so pregnant patients should be given adequate analgesia. Acetaminophen is safe and effective; nonsteroidal anti-inflammatories are given only with the obstetrician's approval because they may adversely affect the fetal environment. Narcotics are generally safe, although hydromorphone and codeine are less preferred.

During pregnancy the maximum recommended dose of radiation exposure is 50 mGy (5 rad). Usually the uterus is outside the field of view for upper extremity procedures and receives an extremely low radiation dose. Abdominal and pelvic computed tomographic (CT) scans deliver doses of 25 mGy. Ultrasound and magnetic resonance imaging offer no known risks. To balance maternal and fetal concerns, it is recommended that conventional radiography be used when possible, ultrasound and magnetic resonance imaging be used for soft tissue imaging, and CT be reserved for essential uses only, with lead shielding during all irradiating procedures.

Conclusions.—Pregnancy is not a contraindication to necessary surgery. If possible, surgery should be delayed until the second trimester. Regional anesthesia is the preferred method of anesthetizing the patient. Acetaminophen is the safest nonnarcotic pain medication. Perioperative narcotic pain control can be achieved using oxycodone. Extremity radiographs and fluoroscopy cause minimal radiation exposure to the fetus and are safe, with CT delivering a substantial higher dose of radiation. It is important that the pregnant patient be managed through a collaboration of efforts from the obstetric, anesthetic, and surgical teams throughout the perioperative and postoperative periods.

▶ This is an excellent, concise review of the operative and perioperative management of the pregnant patient. Bottom line, the most important component of the pregnant patient's case is constant collaboration among the obstetric, anesthetic, and surgical teams at all times. Specific suggestions made in this article are helpful.

D. J. Smith, Jr, MD

Accuracy of Sonographically Guided and Palpation Guided Scaphotrapeziotrapezoid Joint Injections
Smith J, Brault JS, Rizzo M, et al (Mayo Clinic Sports Medicine Ctr, Rochester, MN; Mayo Clinic College of Medicine, Rochester, MN)
J Ultrasound Med 30:1509-1515, 2011

Objectives.—The purpose of this study was to determine and compare the accuracies of sonographically guided and palpation guided scaphotrapeziotrapezoid (STT) joint injections in a cadaveric model.

Methods.—A clinician with 6 years of experience performing sonographically guided procedures injected 1.0 mL of a diluted latex solution into the STT joints of 20 unembalmed cadaveric wrist specimens using a palmar approach. At a minimum of 24 hours after injection, an experienced clinician specializing in hand care completed palpation guided injections in the same specimens using a dorsal approach and 1 mL of a different-colored latex. A fellowship-trained hand surgeon blinded to the injection technique then dissected each specimen to assess injection accuracy. Injections were graded as accurate if the colored latex was found in the STT joint, whereas inaccurate injections resulted in no latex being found in the joint.

Results.—All sonographically guided injections were accurate (100%; 95% confidence interval, 81%−100%), whereas only 80% of palpation guided injections were accurate (95% confidence interval, 61%–99%). Sonographically guided injections were significantly more accurate than palpation guided injections, as determined by the ability to deliver latex into the joint ($P < .05$).

Conclusions.—Sonographic guidance can be used to inject the STT joint with a high degree of accuracy and is more accurate than palpation guidance within the limits of this study design. Clinicians should consider using sonographic guidance to perform STT joint injections when precise intra-articular placement is desired. Further clinical investigation examining the role of sonographically guided STT joint injections in the treatment of patients with radial wrist pain syndromes is warranted.

▶ Scaphotrapeziotrapezoid (STT) arthritis is a common cause of radial wrist pain in the elderly. This article compares the successful placement of latex in the appropriate joint space between a dorsal STT palpation-guided approach and a volar sonographically-guided injection. Both techniques were very reliable, but the sonographically-guided technique was 100% reliable. There are several potential shortcomings of the study, including the use of cadaveric wrists, but the simplicity and accuracy strongly support its adoption as routine.

D. J. Smith, Jr, MD

Predictors of the accuracy of quotation of references in peer-reviewed orthopaedic literature in relation to publications on the scaphoid

Buijze GA, Weening AA, Poolman RW, et al (Massachusetts General Hosp, Boston)
J Bone Joint Surg Br 94-B:276-280, 2012

Using inaccurate quotations can propagate misleading information, which might affect the management of patients. The aim of this study was to determine the predictors of quotation inaccuracy in the peer-reviewed orthopaedic literature related to the scaphoid. We randomly selected 100 papers from ten orthopaedic journals. All references were retrieved in full text when available or otherwise excluded. Two observers independently rated all quotations from the selected papers by comparing the claims made by the authors with the data and expressed opinions of the reference source. A statistical analysis determined which article-related factors were predictors of quotation inaccuracy. The mean total inaccuracy rate of the 3840 verified quotes was 7.6%. There was no correlation between the rate of inaccuracy and the impact factor of the journal. Multivariable analysis identified the journal and the type of study (clinical, biomechanical, methodological, case report or review) as important predictors of the total quotation inaccuracy rate.

We concluded that inaccurate quotations in the peer-reviewed orthopaedic literature related to the scaphoid were common and slightly more so for certain journals and certain study types. Authors, reviewers and editorial staff play an important role in reducing this inaccuracy.

▶ The authors conclude that inaccurate quotations in the peer-reviewed orthopedic literature related to the scaphoid were common (7.6%) and slightly more so for certain journals and certain study types. Substitute any plastic surgery topic for scaphoid, and the conclusion seems equally valid. In fact, the authors note they "are unaware of any reason that assumes significant differences between the specialties of medical literature..." These analyses were relatively new to me but extremely enlightening. They show how incorrect information can easily be perpetuated in the literature. In fact, the authors highlight how a frequently referenced article was misquoted in 63 of 154 articles examined. Their suggestions to improve the accuracy include (1) systematically verify all references against the original documents, (2) be more vigilant and precise in their referencing practices, (3) review their own references fully at least once before publication, and (4) avoid using abstracts (incomplete data) and reviews (indirect references) as references. These should be taken very seriously.

D. J. Smith, Jr, MD

Scaphoid Fractures: What's Hot, What's Not
Geissler WB, Adams JE, Bindra RR, et al (Univ of Mississippi Health Care, Jackson; Univ of Minnesota, Minneapolis; Loyola Univ Health System, Maywood, IL; et al)
J Bone Joint Surg Am 94:169-181, 2012

Fractures of the scaphoid are common injuries. There are several treatment options available, including percutaneous, arthroscopic, and open volar and dorsal approaches. There are advantages and disadvantages associated with each technique, and the surgeon should select what is most comfortable in his or her hands. In addition, for resistant scaphoid nonunions, there are multiple vascularized bone-grafting techniques to obtain union in these difficult fractures.

▶ This is an excellent review of the management of scaphoid fractures as outlined in an instructional course lecture from the American Academy of Orthopedic Surgeons. What is hot in the management of scaphoid fractures over the past 2 decades is the development of percutaneous arthroscopic techniques of scaphoid stabilization that minimize surgical morbidity. Also hot is the substantial improvement in the treatment of difficult scaphoid nonunions with or without deformity. What is not hot is prolonged immobilization for unstable scaphoid fractures when surgical stabilization may have been the best option and complications from an arthroscopic or open procedure that potentially could have been avoided. This is a must read for anyone doing wrist surgery.

D. J. Smith, Jr, MD

Does the Severity of Bilateral Carpal Tunnel Syndrome Influence the Timing of Staged Bilateral Release?

Chin SH, Tom LK, Thomson JG (Yale Univ School of Medicine, New Haven, CT)

Ann Plast Surg 67:30-33, 2011

A retrospective chart analysis was performed of 66 patients with bilateral carpal tunnel syndrome (CTS) who underwent either single endoscopic carpal tunnel release (ECTR) or staged bilateral ECTR to determine the frequency and timing of contralateral surgery.

Bilateral CTS patients with contralateral severe CTS underwent bilateral staged ECTR 86% of the time and the second operation was performed 6 ± 5 weeks after the initial ECTR. Patients with contralateral moderate CTS underwent bilateral staged ECTR 74% of the time with a mean of 11 ± 3 months between operations. Patients with contralateral mild CTS underwent bilateral staged ECTR 20% of the time and averaged 7 ± 3 years between procedures.

For patients with bilateral CTS, the severity of CTS on the contralateral side to the initial release affects both the frequency and timing of the contralateral surgery. This information may be used to establish guidelines for treatment with bilateral simultaneous CTR.

▶ Bilateral carpal tunnel syndrome (CTS) is relatively frequent. Neither the authors nor I initially offered simultaneous release for both hands. On the basis of the review of their treatment of these syndromes, the authors now recommend simultaneous release for bilateral severe CTS and unilateral severe/unilateral moderate severity patients. They are evaluating this treatment prospectively. I predict the results will support their current approach.

D. J. Smith, Jr, MD

The Sensitivity and Specificity of Ultrasound for the Diagnosis of Carpal Tunnel Syndrome: A Meta-analysis

Fowler JR, Gaughan JP, Ilyas AM (Temple Univ Hosp, Philadelphia, PA; Temple Univ School of Medicine, Philadelphia, PA)

Clin Orthop Relat Res 469:1089-1094, 2011

Background.—Carpal tunnel syndrome (CTS) is the most commonly diagnosed compression neuropathy of the upper extremity. Current AAOS recommendations are to obtain a confirmatory electrodiagnostic test in patients for whom surgery is being considered. Ultrasound has emerged as an alternative confirmatory test for CTS; however, its potential role is limited by lack of adequate data for sensitivity and specificity relative to electrodiagnostic testing.

Questions/Purposes.—In this meta-analysis we determined the sensitivity and specificity of ultrasound in the diagnosis of CTS.

Methods.—A PubMed/MEDLINE search identified 323 articles for review. After applying exclusion criteria, 19 articles with a total sample size of 3131 wrists were included for meta-analysis. Three groups were created: a composite of all studies, studies using clinical diagnosis as the reference standard, and studies using electrodiagnostic testing as the reference standard.

Results.—The composite sensitivity and specificity of ultrasound for the diagnosis of CTS, using all studies, were 77.6% (95% CI 71.6–83.6%) and 86.8% (95% CI 78.9–94.8%), respectively.

Conclusions.—The wide variations of sensitivities and specificities reported in the literature have prevented meaningful analysis of ultrasound as either a screening or confirmatory tool in the diagnosis of CTS. The sensitivity and specificity of ultrasound in the diagnosis of CTS are 77.6% and 86.8%, respectively. Although ultrasound may not replace electrodiagnostic testing as the most sensitive and specific test for the diagnosis of CTS given the values reported in this meta-analysis, it may be a feasible alternative to electrodiagnostic testing as the first-line confirmatory test.

Level of Evidence.—Level III, systematic review of Level III studies. See Guidelines for Authors for a complete description of levels of evidence.

▶ I am delighted to see this article. I have never understood the enthusiasm for ultrasound diagnosis of carpal tunnel syndrome. These results confirm to me that there is no place for its use. Why there is some hope for its use in screening is puzzling. These results seem to confirm abandoning its use.

D. J. Smith, Jr, MD

The outcome of carpal tunnel decompression in patients with diabetes mellitus
Jenkins PJ, Duckworth AD, Watts AC, et al (Queen Margaret Hosp, Dunfermline, UK)
J Bone Joint Surg Br 94-B:811-814, 2012

Diabetes mellitus is recognised as a risk factor for carpal tunnel syndrome. The response to treatment is unclear, and may be poorer than in non-diabetic patients. Previous randomised studies of interventions for carpal tunnel syndrome have specifically excluded diabetic patients. The aim of this study was to investigate the epidemiology of carpal tunnel syndrome in diabetic patients, and compare the outcome of carpal tunnel decompression with non-diabetic patients. The primary endpoint was improvement in the QuickDASH score. The prevalence of diabetes mellitus was 11.3% (176 of 1564). Diabetic patients were more likely to have severe neurophysiological findings at presentation. Patients with diabetes had poorer QuickDASH scores at one year post-operatively ($p = 0.028$), although the mean difference was lower than the minimal clinically important difference for this score. After controlling for underlying differences in age and gender, there was no difference between groups in the magnitude of improvement after decompression ($p = 0.481$). Patients with diabetes mellitus can therefore be expected to enjoy a similar improvement in function.

▶ The aim of this study was to investigate the epidemiology of carpal tunnel syndrome (CTS) in diabetic patients and compare the outcome of carpal tunnel decompression (CTD) with that of nondiabetic patients. The outcome of CTD in diabetic patients is unclear, as many larger prospective trials have specifically excluded diabetic patients. This has led to a paucity of evidence supporting CTD for CTS in diabetics. These authors note that after controlling for underlying differences in age and gender, there was no difference between groups in the magnitude of improvement after decompression. The key, though, is to carefully evaluate diabetic patients for additional upper limb pathology. This will be what ultimately determines the success after CTD.

D. J. Smith, Jr, MD

A Tailored Approach to the Surgical Treatment of Cubital Tunnel Syndrome
Keith J, Wollstein R (Univ of Pittsburgh Med Ctr, PA; Veterans Administration of Pittsburgh, PA)
Ann Plast Surg 66:637-639, 2011

Multiple studies have compared the outcome of surgery for cubital tunnel syndrome (CUTS), yet there remains no clear guidelines for treatment. We describe an approach to CUTS that includes tailoring the procedure to the pathology found at surgery. Patients treated surgically were retrospectively reviewed. Following in situ neurolysis, nerve stability within the cubital tunnel was assessed, and the nerve was left in situ, or transposed accordingly. We evaluated demographic information, presenting features, intraoperative and postoperative findings. Statistics included paired t test and logistic regression analysis. A total of 63 patients (standard deviation $= 10.3$ years) were reviewed. Fourteen nerves were transposed (22.5%). Postoperatively, sensation (71%), static 2-point discrimination, and motor strength improved. Grip strength compared with the uninvolved side was 94.8% postoperatively. Overall, 90% of the patients reported improvement in function. Our results compare favorably with other studies. Since CUTS originates from numerous causes, basing the operative plan on intraoperative findings produces excellent results.

▶ The authors present their management of cubital tunnel syndrome (CUTS). Most importantly, they observe that most previous studies assume CUTS is a uniform disease and, therefore, compare standard surgical treatments. These authors use intraoperative findings that select their surgical procedure. Although the numbers are not large enough and the follow-up is not detailed enough, the concept of trying to individualize the procedure to specific findings is important. Their results are encouraging, and a prospective randomized trial will be important.

D. J. Smith, Jr, MD

Painful Nodules and Cords in Dupuytren Disease

von Campe A, Mende K, Omaren H, et al (Kantonsspital Aarau, Tellstrasse, Switzerland)
J Hand Surg 37A:1313-1318, 2012

Purpose.—The etiology of Dupuytren disease is unclear. Pain is seldom described in the literature. Patients are more often disturbed by impaired extension of the fingers. We recently treated a series of patients who had had painful nodules for more than 1 year, and we therefore decided to investigate them for a possible anatomical correlate.

Methods.—Biopsies were taken during surgery from patients with Dupuytren disease and stained to enable detection of neuronal tissue.

Results.—We treated 17 fingers in 10 patients. Intraoperatively, 10 showed tiny nerve branches passing into or crossing the fibrous bands or nodules. Of 13 biopsies, 6 showed nerve fibers embedded in fibrous tissue, 3 showed perineural or intraneural fibrosis or both, and 3 showed true neuromas. Enlarged Pacinian corpuscles were isolated from 1 sample. All patients were pain free after surgery.

Conclusions.—Although Dupuytren disease is generally considered painless, we treated a series of early stage patients with painful disease. Intraoperative inspection and histological examination of tissue samples showed that nerve tissue was involved in all cases. The pain might have been due to local nerve compression by the fibromatosis or the Dupuytren disease itself. We, therefore, suggest that the indication for surgery in Dupuytren disease be extended to painful nodules for more than 1 year, even in the early stages of the disease in the absence of functional deficits, with assessment of tissue samples for histological changes in nerves.

Type of Study/Level of Evidence.—Therapeutic II.

▶ The authors recommend that the indication for surgery in Dupuytren disease be extended to the presence of painful nodules for more than 1 year, even in the early stages of the disease in the absence of functional deficits. Although many of us were taught that Dupuytren disease is not associated with pain, their small sample seems to support this recommendation. I am not prepared to accept this as a blanket recommendation. Caution is still warranted. Any resection in such patients should include assessment for histological changes in nerve fibers.

D. J. Smith, Jr, MD

Cost-Effectiveness of Open Partial Fasciectomy, Needle Aponeurotomy, and Collagenase Injection for Dupuytren Contracture

Chen NC, Shauver MJ, Chung KC (Univ of Michigan Med School, Ann Arbor)
J Hand Surg 36A:1826-1834, 2011

Purpose.—We undertook a cost-utility analysis to compare traditional fasciectomy for Dupuytren with 2 new treatments, needle aponeurotomy and collagenase injection.

Methods.—We constructed an expected-value decision analysis model with an arm representing each treatment. A survey was administered to a cohort of 50 consecutive subjects to determine utilities of different interventions. We conducted multiple sensitivity analyses to assess the impact of varying the rate of disease recurrence in each arm of the analysis as well as the cost of the collagenase injection. The threshold for a cost-effective treatment is based on the traditional willingness-to-pay of $50,000 per quality-adjusted life years (QALY) gained.

Results.—The cost of open partial fasciectomy was $820,114 per QALY gained over no treatment. The cost of needle aponeurotomy was $96,474 per QALY gained versus no treatment. When we performed a sensitivity analysis and set the success rate at 100%, the cost of needle aponeurotomy was $49,631. When needle aponeurotomy was performed without surgical center or anesthesia costs and with reduced hand therapy, the cost was $36,570. When a complete collagenase injection series was priced at $250, the cost was $31,856 per QALY gained. When the injection series was priced at $945, the cost was $49,995 per QALY gained. At the market price of $5,400 per injection, the cost was $166,268 per QALY gained.

Conclusions.—In the current model, open partial fasciectomy is not cost-effective. Needle aponeurotomy is cost-effective if the success rate is high. Collagenase injection is cost-effective when priced under $945.

Type of Study/Level of Evidence.—Economic and Decision Analysis II.

▶ The authors compare the cost-effectiveness of open partial fasciectomy, needle aponeurotomy, and collagenase injection for dupuytren contracture. They used a cost-effectiveness model and analyses that follows the guidelines of the Panel as Cost-effectiveness in Health and Medicine developed by the United States Public Health Service in 1993. These guidelines help ensure consistency among cost-effectiveness analyses. This is not an approach with which many of us are familiar. It will become increasingly important to understand this methodology.

Ultimately, these analyses can guide physicians and patients to arrive at an informed decision in treatment analysis. I would recommend this article to anyone trying to better understand cost-effectiveness.

D. J. Smith, Jr, MD

Nerve injuries sustained during warfare: Part I – Epidemiology
Birch R, Eardley WGP, Ramasamy A, et al (Defence Medicine Rehabilitation Centre, Epsom, UK)
J Bone Joint Surg Br 94-B:523-528, 2012

We describe 261 peripheral nerve injuries sustained in war by 100 consecutive service men and women injured in Iraq and Afghanistan. Their mean age was 26.5 years (18.1 to 42.6), the median interval between injury and first review was 4.2 months (mean 8.4 months (0.36 to 48.49)) and median follow-up was 28.4 months (mean 20.5 months (1.3 to 64.2)).

The nerve lesions were predominantly focal prolonged conduction block/neurapraxia in 116 (45%), axonotmesis in 92 (35%) and neurotmesis in 53 (20%) and were evenly distributed between the upper and the lower limbs. Explosions accounted for 164 (63%): 213 (82%) nerve injuries were associated with open wounds. Two or more main nerves were injured in 70 patients. The ulnar, common peroneal and tibial nerves were most commonly injured. In 69 patients there was a vascular injury, fracture, or both at the level of the nerve lesion. Major tissue loss was present in 50 patients: amputation of at least one limb was needed in 18. A total of 36 patients continued in severe neuropathic pain.

This paper outlines the methods used in the assessment of these injuries and provides information about the depth and distribution of the nerve lesions, their associated injuries and neuropathic pain syndromes.

▶ Between 2005 and 2010, all United Kingdom Service personnel with peripheral nerve injuries (PNI) from ballistic trauma were examined in the War Nerve Injury Clinic at the Defense Medical Rehabilitation Center. This article and part II with the same title detail subgroup analysis of these patients. This article, epidemiology, outlines the methods used in the assessment of these injuries and provides information about the depth and distribution of the nerve lesions, their associated injuries, and neuropathic pain syndromes. Part II describes outcomes.[1] Of interest, there was no difference in the outcomes of penetrating inside wounds and those caused by explosions. War is clearly horrific. Hopefully, articles and analyses such as this will at least help us with future treatments.

D. J. Smith, Jr, MD

Reference

1. Birch R, Misra P, Stewart MP, et al. Nerve injuries sustained during warfare: part II: outcomes. *J Bone Joint Surg Br.* 2012;94-B:529-535.

Nerve injuries sustained during warfare: Part II: Outcomes
Birch R, Eardley WGP, Ramasamy A, et al (Defence Med Rehabilitation Centre, Epsom, UK)
J Bone Joint Surg Br 94-B:529-535, 2012

The outcomes of 261 nerve injuries in 100 patients were graded good in 173 cases (66%), fair in 70 (26.8%) and poor in 18 (6.9%) at the final review (median 28.4 months (1.3 to 64.2)). The initial grades for the 42 sutures and graft were 11 good, 14 fair and 17 poor. After subsequent revision repairs in seven, neurolyses in 11 and free vascularised fasciocutaneous flaps in 11, the final grades were 15 good, 18 fair and nine poor. Pain was relieved in 30 of 36 patients by nerve repair, revision of repair or neurolysis, and flaps when indicated. The difference in outcome between penetrating missile wounds and those caused by explosions was not statistically significant; in the latter group the onset of recovery from focal conduction block was delayed (mean

4.7 months (2.5 to 10.2) *vs* 3.8 months (0.6 to 6); $p = 0.0001$). A total of 42 patients (47 lower limbs) presented with an insensate foot. By final review (mean 27.4 months (20 to 36)) plantar sensation was good in 26 limbs (55%), fair in 16 (34%) and poor in five (11%). Nine patients returned to full military duties, 18 to restricted duties, 30 to sedentary work, and 43 were discharged from military service. Effective rehabilitation must be early, integrated and vigorous. The responsible surgeons must be firmly embedded in the process, at times exerting leadership.

▶ Between 2005 and 2010, all United Kingdom Service personnel with peripheral nerve injuries (PNI) from ballistic trauma were examined in the War Nerve Injury Clinic at the Defense Medical Rehabilitation Center. This article and part I[1] with the same title detail subgroup analysis of these patients. Part I of this article, epidemiology, outlines the methods used in the assessment of these injuries and provides information about the depth and distribution of the nerve lesions, their associated injuries, and neuropathic pain syndromes. This article, part II, describes outcomes. Of interest, there was no difference in the outcomes of penetrating inside wounds and those caused by explosions. War is clearly horrific. Hopefully, articles and analyses such as this will help us with future treatments.

D. J. Smith, Jr, MD

Reference

1. Birch R, Misra P, Stewart MP, et al. Nerve injuries sustained during warfare: part I—Epidemiology. *J Bone Joint Surg Br.* 2012;94:523-528.

Outcome models in peripheral nerve repair: time for a reappraisal or for a novel?
Galanakos SP, Zoubos AB, Johnson EO, et al (Univ of Athens, Greece)
Microsurgery 32:326-333, 2012

Peripheral nerve injuries are still underestimated. The complexity of assessment of outcome after nerve injury and repair has been described by many authors. Furthermore, the outcome is influenced by several factors that depend on mechanisms in the peripheral as well as the central nervous system. Appropriate formulation of a global accepted postoperative clinical protocol for peripheral nerve repair in the upper extremity remains a subject of debate. The purpose of this review is to detail the current concepts of methods of evaluation after peripheral nerves repair. Finally, we discuss the most crucial factors that determine the final hand function and we consider the challenges that need to be addressed to create a realistic clinical protocol that reflects a prognostic importance.

▶ This review details the current concepts of evaluation after peripheral nerve repair. Because of the difficulty ascertaining the success of a nerve repair, many have suggested formulation of a realistic prognostic score based on the results of published survey data. This article does not tackle this formulation but is an excellent and thorough review of evaluation methods available with their strengths and weaknesses. This is a must-read review for those interested in comprehensively following their peripheral nerve injury patients.

D. J. Smith, Jr, MD

Processed nerve allografts for peripheral nerve reconstruction: a multicenter study of utilization and outcomes in sensory, mixed, and motor nerve reconstructions
Brooks DN, Weber RV, Chao JD, et al (The Buncke Clinic, San Francisco, CA; Albert Einstein College of Medicine, Bronx, NY; Albany Med College, NY; et al)
Microsurgery 32:1-14, 2012

Purpose.—As alternatives to autograft become more conventional, clinical outcomes data on their effectiveness in restoring meaningful function is essential. In this study we report on the outcomes from a multicenter study on processed nerve allografts (Avance® Nerve Graft, AxoGen, Inc).

Patients and Methods.—Twelve sites with 25 surgeons contributed data from 132 individual nerve injuries. Data was analyzed to determine the safety and efficacy of the nerve allograft. Sufficient data for efficacy analysis were reported in 76 injuries (49 sensory, 18 mixed, and 9 motor nerves). The mean age was 41 ± 17 (18−86) years. The mean graft length was 22 ± 11 (5−50) mm. Subgroup analysis was performed to determine the relationship to factors known to influence outcomes of nerve repair such as nerve type, gap length, patient age, time to repair, age of injury, and mechanism of injury.

Results.—Meaningful recovery was reported in 87% of the repairs reporting quantitative data. Subgroup analysis demonstrated consistency, showing no significant differences with regard to recovery outcomes between the groups ($P > 0.05$ Fisher's Exact Test). No graft related adverse experiences were reported and a 5% revision rate was observed.

Conclusion.—Processed nerve allografts performed well and were found to be safe and effective in sensory, mixed and motor nerve defects between 5 and 50 mm. The outcomes for safety and meaningful recovery observed in this study compare favorably to those reported in the literature for nerve autograft and are higher than those reported for nerve conduits.

▶ The authors present a multicenter trial of nerve allografts, which is certainly one of the largest such studies to date. They report that processed nerve allografts are a safe and effective alternative for nerve reconstruction with meaningful recovery reported in 87.3% of cases reporting quantitative data. Subgroup analysis also shows that these allografts provide functional recovery in sensory, missed, and motor nerve injuries in gaps up to 50 mm. Obviously, there is the benefit of no donor site morbidity and shorter operating times. The authors make a good case for the use of nerve allografts, but it will be important to follow up with this series longitudinally to be sure there is no deterioration in their results.

D. J. Smith, Jr, MD

FDA approved guidance conduits and wraps for peripheral nerve injury: A review of materials and efficacy
Kehoe S, Zhang XF, Boyd D (Dalhousie Univ, Halifax, Canada; Cork Inst of Technology, Ireland)
Injury 43:553-572, 2012

Several nerve guidance conduits (NGCs) and nerve protectant wraps are approved by the US Food and Drug Administration (FDA) for clinical use in peripheral nerve repair. These devices cover a wide range of natural and synthetic materials, which may or may not be resorbable. This review consolidates the data pertaining to all FDA approved materials into a single reference, which emphasizes material composition alongside pre-clinical and clinical safety and efficacy (where possible). This article also summarizes the key advantages and limitations for each material as noted in the literature (with respect to the indication considered). In this context, this review provides a comprehensive reference for clinicians which may facilitate optimal material/device selection for peripheral nerve repair. For materials scientists, this review highlights predicate devices and evaluation methodologies, offering an insight into current deficiencies associated with state-of-the-art materials and may help direct new technology developments and evaluation methodologies thereof.

▶ Since 1995, 11 devices (several nerve guidance conduits and nerve protective wraps) have been approved by the US Food and Drug Administration (FDA) for the repair of peripheral nerve injuries. These devices cover a wide range of natural and synthetic materials, which may or may not be resorbable. The authors consolidate the data pertaining to all FDA-approved materials emphasizing material composition as well as preclinical and clinical safety and efficacy (where possible). They also summarize the key advantages and limitations for each material as noted in the literature (with respect to the indication considered). The article is a comprehensive reference. For those using these devices, this is an excellent review. For those not familiar with them, this is an excellent guide to when and which ones may be most helpful.

D. J. Smith, Jr, MD

A Systematic Review of the Outcomes of Replantation of Distal Digital Amputation

Sebastin SJ, Chung KC (Natl Univ Health System, Singapore; Univ of Michigan Health System, Ann Arbor)
Plast Reconstr Surg 128:723-737, 2011

Background.—The aim of this study was to conduct a systematic review of the English literature on replantation of distal digital amputations to provide the best evidence of survival rates and functional outcomes.

Methods.—A MEDLINE search using "digit," "finger," "thumb," and "replantation" as keywords and limited to humans and English-language articles identified 1297 studies. Studies were included in the review if they (1) present primary data, (2) report five or more single or multiple distal replantations, and (3) present survival rates. Additional data extracted from the studies meeting the inclusion criteria included demographic information, nature and level of amputation, venous outflow technique, nerve repair, recovery of sensibility, range of motion, return to work, and complications.

Results.—Thirty studies representing 2273 distal replantations met the inclusion criteria. The mean survival rate was 86 percent. There was no difference in survival between zone I and zone II replantations (Tamai classification). There was a significant difference in survival between replantation of clean-cut versus the more crushed amputations (crush-cut and crush-avulsion). The repair of a vein improved survival in both zone I and zone II replantation. The mean two-point discrimination was 7 mm ($n = 220$), and 98 percent returned to work ($n = 98$). Complications included pulp atrophy in 14 percent of patients ($n = 639$) and nail deformity in 23 percent ($n = 653$).

Conclusions.—The common perception that distal replantation is associated with little functional gain is not based on scientific evidence. This systematic review showed a high success rate and good functional outcomes following distal digital replantation.

Clinical Question/Level of Evidence.—Therapeutic, IV.

▶ Once again, Dr Chung and his group have put together an excellent study leading us to better evidenced-based practice. This time, they reviewed the outcomes of replantation of distal digital amputations. There are a number of interesting findings. To begin with, the common perception that distal replantation is associated with little functional gain is not based on scientific evidence. Their systematic review showed a high success rate and good functional outcomes after distal digital replantation.

They drill down on a number of interesting trends. The vast majority of these cases were performed in Asia, where the surgeons cite Confucian moral values and a greater emphasis on maintaining body integrity and physical appearance as a reason for performing these procedures. They further make the case for specialized centers in the United States. This is a must read for anyone involved in the care of these patients.

D. J. Smith, Jr, MD

Limb Transplantation and Targeted Reinnervation: A Practical Comparison

Agnew SP, Ko J, De La Garza M, et al (Northwestern Memorial Hosp, Chicago, IL; et al)
J Reconstr Microsurg 28:63-68, 2012

Limb transplantation and targeted reinnervation are complimentary but very different approaches for restoring function to an upper limb amputee. This article reviews the advantages and limitations of both of these procedures, and highlights the reconstructive obstacles in the treatment of upper limb amputees.

▶ The authors compare upper limb transplantation with targeted reinnervation. They present a nice overview of both. Most importantly, they compare the 2 methods level by level. This is very enlightening for those who have not kept up with the advances in targeted reinnervation. Also important is understanding that these are complementary, not competitive, procedures at this time.

D. J. Smith, Jr, MD

Update on Advances in Upper Extremity Prosthetics

Behrend C, Reizner W, Marchessault JA, et al (Univ of Rochester Med Ctr, NY; Walter Reed Army Med Ctr, Washington, DC)
J Hand Surg 36A:1711-1717, 2011

Upper extremity amputations are common. Fortunately, most of these involve loss of only a finger or portion thereof. Hand and upper limb surgeons are best suited to lead the team and help these patients following these injuries. Proximal amputations can be devastating for the patient, but recent prosthetic advances have helped many patients lead a better life and, often, return to activities they were involved in before their amputation. The purpose of this article is to review the current prostheses available for upper extremity amputees.

▶ A full understanding of the current status of upper extremity prosthetics is important. This article is clear, with enough detail to be helpful and not so much as to be burdensome. Rejection rates of the use of prostheses may approach 40% and increase as the amputation level moves toward the shoulder. Early fitting, within 30 days, is stressed. This article provides an important review for any surgeon working with upper extremity trauma.

D. J. Smith, Jr, MD

Assessing the Impact of Antibiotic Prophylaxis in Outpatient Elective Hand Surgery: A Single-Center, Retrospective Review of 8,850 Cases

Bykowski MR, Sivak WN, Cray J, et al (Dept of Plastic and Reconstructive Surgery, Pittsburgh, PA; Hand and Upper Extremity Ctr, Wexford, PA; Johns Hopkins Univ School of Medicine, Baltimore, MD)
J Hand Surg 36A:1741-1747, 2011

Purpose.—Prophylactic antibiotics have been shown to prevent surgical site infection (SSI) after some gastrointestinal, orthopedic, and plastic surgical procedures, but their efficacy in clean, elective hand surgery is unclear. Our aims were to assess the efficacy of preoperative antibiotics in preventing SSI after clean, elective hand surgery, and to identify potential risk factors for SSI.

Methods.—We queried the database from an outpatient surgical center by Current Procedural Terminology code to identify patients who underwent elective hand surgery. For each medical record, we collected patient demographics and characteristics along with preoperative, intraoperative, and postoperative management details. The primary outcome of this study was SSI, and secondary outcomes were wound dehiscence and suture granuloma.

Results.—From October 2000 through October 2008, 8,850 patient records met our inclusion criteria. The overall SSI rate was 0.35%, with an average patient follow-up duration of 79 days. The SSI rates did not significantly differ between patients receiving antibiotics (0.54%; 2,755 patients) and those who did not (0.26%; 6,095 patients). Surgical site infection was associated with smoking status, diabetes mellitus, and longer procedure length irrespective of antibiotic use. Subgroup analysis revealed that prophylactic antibiotics did not prevent SSI in male patients, smokers, or diabetics, or for procedure length less than 30 minutes, 30 to 60 minutes, and greater than 60 minutes.

Conclusions.—Prophylactic antibiotic administration does not reduce the incidence of SSI after clean, elective hand surgery in an outpatient population. Moreover, subgroup analysis revealed that prophylactic antibiotics did not reduce the frequency of SSI among patients who were found to be at higher risk in this study. We identified 3 factors associated with the development of SSI in our study: diabetes mellitus status, procedure length, and smoking status. Given the potential harmful complications associated with antibiotic use and the lack of evidence that prophylactic antibiotics prevent SSIs, we conclude that antibiotics should not be routinely administered to patients who undergo clean, elective hand surgery.

Type of Study/Level of Evidence.—Therapeutic III.

▶ The authors assess the efficacy of preoperative antibiotics in preventing surgical site infection (SSI) after clean, elective hand surgery and to identify potential risk factors for SSI. They show prophylactic antibiotic administration does not reduce the incidence of SSI after clean, elective hand surgery in an outpatient population. Moreover, subgroup analysis revealed that prophylactic antibiotics did not reduce the frequency of SSI among patients who were found to be at higher risk in this study. They identified 3 factors associated with the development of SSI in our study: diabetes mellitus status, procedure length, and smoking status. Given the potential harmful complications associated with antibiotic use and the lack of evidence that prophylactic antibiotics prevent SSIs, they conclude that antibiotics should not be routinely administered to patients who undergo clean, elective hand surgery. This should strongly be considered as standard of care.

D. J. Smith, Jr, MD

Opioid Consumption Following Outpatient Upper Extremity Surgery

Rodgers J, Cunningham K, Fitzgerald K, et al (Des Moines Orthopaedic Surgeons and Des Moines Univ, IA)
J Hand Surg 37A:645-650, 2012

Purpose.—After elective outpatient upper extremity surgery, patients' need for opioid analgesic medication may be considerably less than typically dispensed. Our goal for this study was to evaluate pain control and quantify the amount of leftover pain medication.

Methods.—We recruited patients scheduled for elective outpatient upper extremity surgery, who met the inclusion criteria, to participate in a phone interview 7 to 14 days after surgery. Information collected included age, gender, procedure performed, analgesic medication and regimen prescribed, satisfaction with pain control, number of tablets remaining, reasons for not taking medication, other analgesic medications used, payer classification, and any adverse drug reactions.

Results.—A total of 287 eligible subjects consented to participate. Of these, 36 patients failed phone contact and 1 patient canceled surgery, which left 250 patients who completed the study. Oxycodone, hydrocodone, and propoxyphene accounted for over 95% of the prescription medications, with adequate pain control reported by 230 (92%) patients. Patients most frequently received 30 pills. Patients undergoing bone procedures reported the highest medication use (14 pills), whereas patients undergoing soft tissue procedures reported the lowest use (9 pills). Over half of the subjects reported taking the opioid medication for 2 days or less. Medicare patients consumed significantly less medication (7 pills, $P < .05$) than patients covered by all other types of insurance. Overall, patients consumed a mean of 10 opioid pills, whereas 19 pills per subject were reported unused, which resulted in 4,639 leftover tablets for the entire cohort.

Conclusions.—Our data show that excess opioid analgesics are made available after elective upper extremity surgery and could potentially become a source for diversion. A prescription of 30 opioid pills for outpatient surgery appears excessive and unnecessary, especially for soft tissue procedures of the hand and wrist.

Type of Study/Level of Evidence.—Prognostic I.

▶ This study evaluates the patient use of opioid analgesics after elective upper extremity surgery. It determined that patients need much less pain medicine than typically dispensed. This is ironic in view of the increased emphasis on pain management. There are a number of shortcomings to the study, including no control for previous surgery, type of anesthesia, and postoperative complications. But all in all, the study challenges us to review our prescribing patterns. It appears that a large amount of pain medicine is unnecessarily dispensed. Significant cost savings may be realized without jeopardizing patient care.

D. J. Smith, Jr, MD

Epinephrine and Hand Surgery
Mann T, Hammert WC (Univ of Rochester Med Ctr, NY)
J Hand Surg 37A:1254-1256, 2012

Background.—Traditional concern for the use of epinephrine in the fingers is founded on 21 cases of digital necrosis reported after injection with a local anesthetic with epinephrine. In all cases, which usually occurred before 1950, procaine was used, which may have been expired, giving it a toxically low pH. Phentolamine readily reverses the effects of epinephrine in the fingers. The evidence concerning links between the use of epinephrine and the occurrence of digital necrosis was reviewed.

Evidence Review.—No finger necrosis has been reported in connection with the use of lidocaine plus epinephrine. Several case reports and case series note patients who have accidentally injected fingers with epinephrine 100 times more concentrated than what is found in lidocaine-epinephrine mixtures, often while using epinephrine auto-injectors. Even when these patients were not treated, no reports of digital necrosis or other permanent harmful outcomes were found. A prospective review of over 1300 cases of digital blocks uncovered no cases of digital necrosis, no need for phentolamine rescue, and no long-term ill effects. It should be noted, however, that little evidence indicates that the augmentation of digital blocks with epinephrine produces better outcomes.

Analysis.—Since there is no evidence of finger necrosis occurring in connection with the use of epinephrine in digital blocks, it should be considered safe. Research is needed to assess whether there are links between the use of epinephrine in digital blocks and effects on patient satisfaction, complications, and cost.

Conclusions.—Lidocaine plus epinephrine is widely used in the belief that the epinephrine improves hemostasis, diminishes the need for tourniquet use and sedation, and lowers costs associated with complications. If the patient is not sedated, the surgeon can perform intraoperative assessment of active range of motion, which can benefit flexor tendon repair, tendolysis, and tendon transfer procedures. Using epinephrine also may increase the duration of the analgesic effect. Caution should be exercised for patients with known peripheral vascular disease; diabetes; Raynaud phenomenon; Berger's disease; the syndrome of calcinosis, Raynaud phenomenon, esophageal dysmotility, sclerodactyly, and telangiectasia; and other conditions associated with digital perfusion.

▶ Traditional concern regarding the use of epinephrine in the fingers is based on 21 reported cases of digital necrosis after being injected with a local anesthetic with epinephrine. Most occurred before 1950 and all use procaine. In the world literature, no cases of finger necrosis have been reported after the use of lidocaine with epinephrine. The use of epinephrine with local anesthesia is becoming more commonplace in hand surgery. It also improves hemostasis and decreases the need for tourniquet use and sedation. This is an excellent review of the current use of epinephrine with local anesthesia. We must be careful to monitor closely as the use increases.

D. J. Smith, Jr, MD

Exploring the Application of Stem Cells in Tendon Repair and Regeneration
Ahmad Z, Wardale J, Brooks R, et al (Addenbrooke's Hosp, Cambridge, England, UK; Royal Liverpool Univ Hosp, England, UK)
Arthroscopy 28:1018-1029, 2012

Purpose.—To conduct a systematic review of the current evidence for the effects of stem cells on tendon healing in preclinical studies and human studies.

Methods.—A systematic search of the PubMed, CINAHL (Cumulative Index to Nursing and Allied Health Literature), Cochrane, and Embase databases was performed for stem cells and tendons with their associated terminology. Data validity was assessed, and data were collected on the outcomes of trials.

Results.—A total of 27 preclinical studies and 5 clinical studies met the inclusion criteria. Preclinical studies have shown that stem cells are able to survive and differentiate into tendon cells when placed into a new tendon environment, leading to regeneration and biomechanical benefit to the tendon. Studies have been reported showing that stem cell therapy can be enhanced by molecular signaling adjunct, mechanical stimulation of cells, and the use of augmentation delivery devices. Studies have also shown alternatives to the standard method of bone marrow—derived mesenchymal stem cell therapy. Of the 5 human studies, only 1 was a randomized controlled trial, which showed that skin-derived tendon cells had a greater clinical benefit than autologous plasma. One cohort study showed the benefit of stem cells in rotator cuff tears and another in lateral epicondylitis. Two of the human studies showed how stem cells were successfully extracted from the humerus and, when tagged with insulin, became tendon cells.

Conclusions.—The current evidence shows that stem cells can have a positive effect on tendon healing. This is most likely because stem cells have regeneration potential, producing tissue that is similar to the preinjury state, but the results can be variable. The use of adjuncts such as molecular signaling, mechanical stimulation, and augmentation devices can potentially enhance stem cell therapy. Initial clinical trials are promising, with adjuncts for stem cell therapy in development.

Level of Evidence.—Level IV, systematic review of Level II-IV studies.

▶ The authors summarized publications detailing the in vitro, in vivo, and clinical findings of stem cell therapy in tendons. This has shown that stem cells in tendons can increase collagen fiber density, enhance tissue architecture, and restore a nearly normal tendon—bone interface. Studies have shown that the biomechanical benefit of stem cells can be seen if the study is followed up over a longer period.

Stem cells can have a positive effect on tendon healing. This is most likely because stem cells have regeneration potential, producing tissue that is similar to the preinjury state, but the results can be variable. The use of adjuncts such as molecular signaling, mechanical stimulation, and augmentation devices can potentially enhance stem cell therapy. Initial clinical trials are promising, with adjuncts for stem cell therapy in development. The authors present a very complete, comprehensive review of stem cell therapy in tendon healing. This is an excellent primer for those who are looking to understand the upcoming advancements in tendon healing.

D. J. Smith, Jr, MD

Conflicts of Interest With the Hand Surgeon's Relationship With Industry
Delsignore JL, Goodman MJ (Univ of Rochester School of Medicine, NY; Salem Orthopaedic Surgeons, MA)
J Hand Surg 37:179-183, 2012

Many advances in hand surgery have been supported and enabled by the integral relationship that exists between the profession of hand surgery and industry. This relationship takes many forms, including medical education, development of new technology and methodology, research, and opportunities for patient education. As with all of these endeavors, the primary focus of both the physician and industry must be the care of the patient. When a collaborative relationship exists between physicians and industry, a conflict of interest is present and must be recognized as such and managed to avoid any detriment to patient care. Although the hand surgeon, the patient, and industry share the common interest of advancement of patient care, there does exist real and potential conflicts of interest, which are unavoidable, but not necessarily undesirable. Multiple guidelines exist to govern relationships between industry and physicians. The cooperative relationship between the physician and industry is not only helpful, but it can be critical to the advancement of and innovations in patient care. When properly managed, collaboration between the physician and industry can effectively achieve the common goal of serving the best interest of the patient.

▶ This article provides an excellent overview of the potential conflicts of interests in hand surgeons' relationships with industry. As a plastic surgeon, I am disappointed that almost the entire article focuses on the orthopedic approach. American Society of Plastic Surgeons is mentioned only once. Despite that, any review of conflicts of interest is helpful.

D. J. Smith, Jr, MD

5 Aesthetic

General

Screening Tools for Body Dysmorphic Disorder in a Cosmetic Surgery Setting

Picavet V, Gabriëls L, Jorissen M, et al (Univ Hosps Leuven, Belgium)
Laryngoscope 121:2535-2541, 2011

Objectives/Hypothesis.—Body dysmorphic disorder (BDD) is a well-established psychiatric disorder characterized by a marked, distressing, and impairing preoccupation with an imagined or slight defect in appearance. Despite the growing interest in and awareness of aesthetic surgeons for BDD, diagnosing BDD during a preoperative consultation remains challenging. This review provides an overview of the existing screening tools for BDD and assesses their quality and feasibility in an aesthetic surgery population.

Study Design.—Systematic review.

Methods.—An electronic bibliographic search was conducted to identify all screening tools for BDD in a cosmetic setting. We investigated their development and validation processes and investigated whether the screening tool had a predictive value on subjective outcomes after treatment.

Results.—We identified six different screening tools for BDD in a cosmetic setting. Only two of them were validated in a cosmetic dermatology setting: the Body Dysmorphic Disorder Questionnaire—Dermatology Version (BDDQ-DV) and the Dysmorphic Concern Questionnaire (DCQ). Outside the dermatologic surgery setting, no screening tools were validated. For the BDDQ-DV, no influence on subjective outcome after cosmetic treatment was found.

Conclusions.—The limited availability of good screening tools for BDD in patients seeking aesthetic surgery stands in remarkable contrast to the estimated high prevalence of BDD in this setting. Among the currently used screening tools, the BDDQ-DV and the DCQ seem the most suitable for further research on prevalence of BDD in cosmetic surgery and the impact of BDD on treatment outcome.

▶ Not long ago, body dysmorphic disorder (BDD) was thought uncommon and estimated by plastic surgeons to be around 2% of patients seen for primary cosmetic surgery. Newer studies estimate the prevalence of BDD in the general population to be between 0.7% and 7%, and rates of up to 53.6% have been reported in a cosmetic surgery setting. It is likely that most surgeons underestimate the prevalence of BDD in their patients. Almost no patients with BDD benefit from cosmetic surgery, and most show a low degree of satisfaction, a deterioration of BDD symptoms, and even become aggressive and violent toward themselves and/or their surgeon. There is consensus that BDD should be a contraindication for cosmetic treatments.

Unfortunately, the currently available psychometric tests for diagnosing and assessing the severity of BDD are difficult to apply and interpret and have not been validated in a plastic surgery population. Plastic surgeons and their staff must therefore remain more vigilant and proactive in considering BDD in their patients. Empowering the office staff to look for signs of BDD and having a good relationship with a mental health professional with an interest in BDD may help identify these patients before a futile cosmetic treatment is performed.

K. A. Gutowski, MD

Back to Basics: Understanding the Terminology Associated With Light- and Energy-Based Technology

Kulick MI (Plastic Surgeon in Private Practice in San Francisco, CA)
Aesthet Surg J 31:984-986, 2011

Background.—Among the aesthetic treatment alternatives are light- and energy-based devices used to accomplish hair reduction, vascular and pigmentation corrections, contour improvements for fat deposits, and non-surgical wrinkle reduction. To choose the most appropriate option, clinicians rely on published studies, manufacturers' presentations, and colleagues' comments. However, the terms used in reporting data and marketing devices need clarification, especially those used to describe procedures, techniques, and results. The Light- and Energy-Based Therapies Subcommittee of the American Society for Aesthetic Plastic Surgery (ASAPS) identified terms used in promoting products, most specifically those related to the recovery process. The list will be provided to manufacturers for incorporation in marketing efforts. The terms clarified and other committee recommendations were discussed.

Terms.—Terms approved by the subcommittee and ASAPS board were downtime, bruising, redness, swelling, and pain. *Downtime* is the expected time before a patient can resume normal activities. Essentially no downtime means less than 24 hours, minimal downtime 24 to 72 hours, moderate downtime 3 to 7 days, and significant downtime over 7 days. *Bruising* is ecchymosis visible on the skin when no concealer is used. Essentially no bruising means no ecchymosis but allows for some immediate skin tone change. Minimal bruising resolves in less than 1 week, moderate in 1 to 2 weeks, and significant in more than 2 weeks. *Redness* is increased red quality to the skin (hyperemia) without concealer applied. Essentially none means the skin returns to normal (pretreatment or improved) coloring in less than 24 hours, but allows for some immediate skin tone change. Minimal hyperemia resolves in 1 to 3 days, moderate in 4 to 7 days, and significant in more than 7 days. *Swelling* refers to obvious swelling in the treated areas. Essentially none means swelling resolving in less than 3 days, minimal in 3 to 7 days, moderate in 8 to 14 days, and significant in more than 14 days. *Pain* is discomfort associated with treatment. If there is essentially none, no pretreatment medication, local anesthesia during treatment, or posttreatment intervention is needed, although over-the-counter medications may be used. Minimal pain requires pretreatment oral medications (prescribed agents), topical agents and/or skin cooling during treatment, and/or posttreatment prescriptions. Moderate is the same as minimal pain plus pretreatment local anesthesia to achieve results. Significant pain is the same as minimal pain with either pretreatment intravenous sedation or general anesthesia required to obtain the desired results.

Added Recommendations.—Photography should also be standardized, specifically including lighting and patient positioning. Pretreatment photographs should be labeled with the patient's age and device name and posttreatment photographs should show the number of treatments received, any other modalities used, and length of time after final treatment that the patient is shown.

Conclusions.—More terms will be added as the committee develops a full and comprehensive nomenclature. If manufacturers choose to adopt these recommendations, the acceptance and/or adoption of their devices will be facilitated, with physicians able to better understand claims and compare. Companies that abide by these recommendations will be acknowledged at the ASAPS annual meeting.

▶ When faced with investing in, or trying, new technologies, each surgeon hopes to have an objective measurement of what type of outcome can be achieved and the recovery period a patient can expect. Patients who receive directed marketing about the advantages of the latest laser therapies may unrealistically expect superior results with little or no recovery. The American Society for Aesthetic Plastic Surgery now offers a standardized use of terms and definitions for light- and energy-based therapies. This consensus document will be offered to aesthetic industry manufacturers to encourage the standardized use of definitions in their marketing material. Topics include the following:

- Standardized pretreatment and posttreatment photography with attached patient demographics and specific treatment details
- A 4-level grading scale for each category of downtime, bruising, redness, swelling, and pain
- Additional potentially confusing terms will be added in the future to develop standardized nomenclature.

Plastic surgeons should start asking their appropriate product representatives to use this classification system when showing marketing material. Furthermore, the grading scales can be used with patients to help them understand the time needed for recovery and for planning their downtime after treatment.

K. A. Gutowski, MD

Epidural Anesthesia as a Thromboembolic Prophylaxis Modality in Plastic Surgery

Hafezi F, Naghibzadeh B, Nouhi AH, et al (Tehran Univ of Med Sciences, Zaferanieh, Iran; Private Practice, Tehran, Iran; et al)

Aesthet Surg J 31:821-824, 2011

Background.—Epidural anesthesia (EA) is known to reduce postoperative thromboembolic complications, but the mechanisms are poorly understood. Review of the literature revealed no reports about the ability of epidural anesthesia (EA) to reduce the risk of venous thromboembolism (VTE) in abdominal contouring surgery and/or liposuction. Most medical publications in this field are based on orthopedic cases.

Objectives.—The authors investigate the hypothesis that the differential nerve-blocking effect of bupivacaine, which spares motor function and permits leg movement during the operation, is the most important mechanism by which EA prevents thromboembolism.

Methods.—From June 1992 to August 1995, 24 cases of abdominoplasty were performed under general anesthesia (Group 1). From September 1995 to December 2009, 371 cases of concurrent abdominoplasty and liposuction were performed under EA (Group 2). Eighteen cases (4.8%) from Group 2 were ultimately excluded from the study because of unsuccessful EA. All surgeries were performed by the senior author (FH).

Results.—One thromboembolic event (pulmonary embolism [PE]) occurred in Group 1 (4%). No cases of deep vein thrombosis (DVT) or PE occurred among Group 2 patients.

Conclusions.—Together, differential epidural nerve blocks and purposeful intraoperative movement of lower-limb muscles represent an effective prophylactic mechanism that may prevent devastating DVT and resultant PE.

▶ Avoiding general anesthesia in abdominoplasty to decrease venous thromboembolism risk should be considered in appropriate patients. While epidural anesthesia may be useful in these cases, it may not be practical for many surgeons. In this series, there was a 5% epidural failure rate that required conversion to general anesthesia. In many outpatient or office-based surgery facilities, epidural anesthesia may not be as reliable due to the anesthesiologists' skills and experience. Epidural anesthesia has its own risks and potential complications, which need to be considered. Perhaps a better option is using tumescent fluid infiltration and intravenous anesthesia supervised by a nurse anesthetist or anesthesiologist and thereby avoiding the need of inhalational gas anesthesia.

K. A. Gutowski, MD

Aprepitant plus Ondansetron Compared with Ondansetron Alone in Reducing Postoperative Nausea and Vomiting in Ambulatory Patients Undergoing Plastic Surgery

Vallejo MC, Phelps AL, Ibinson JW, et al (Univ of Pittsburgh Med Ctr, PA; Univ of Pittsburgh Med Ctr Veterans Affair Med Ctr, PA; Univ of Pittsburgh Med Ctr St Margaret Hosp, PA; et al)
Plast Reconstr Surg 129:519-526, 2012

Background.—Postoperative nausea and vomiting is a major challenge in the perioperative setting. The incidence can be as high as 80 percent, and the majority of the symptoms among outpatients occur after discharge. This study evaluated the efficacy of a neurokinin-1 receptor antagonist (aprepitant) in reducing postoperative symptoms for up to 48 hours in patients undergoing outpatient plastic surgery.

Methods.—A prospective, double-blinded, randomized, two-arm evaluation of 150 ambulatory plastic surgery patients receiving a standardized general anesthetic, including postoperative nausea and vomiting prophylaxis with ondansetron and either aprepitant or placebo, was performed. The main outcome measures were the occurrence of vomiting and the severity of nausea for up to 48 hours postoperatively.

Results.—Overall, 9.3 percent of patients who received aprepitant versus 29.7 percent in group B had vomiting, with the majority of vomiting episodes occurring after hospital discharge. The Kaplan-Meier plot of the hazards of vomiting revealed an increased incidence of emesis in patients receiving ondansetron alone compared with the combination of ondansetron and aprepitant ($p = 0.006$). The incidence of nausea was not significantly different in the two groups. Severity of nausea, however, was significantly higher in those receiving ondansetron alone compared with those receiving ondansetron and aprepitant, as measured by a peak nausea score ($p = 0.014$) and by multivariate analysis of variance results comparing repeated verbal rating scale scores over 48 hours after surgery ($p = 0.024$).

Conclusion.—In patients undergoing plastic surgery, the addition of aprepitant to ondansetron significantly decreases postoperative vomiting rates and nausea severity for up to 48 hours postoperatively.

Clinical Question/Level of Evidence.—Therapeutic, II.

▶ Aprepitant is a neurokinin-1 receptor antagonist that acts by blocking the binding of substance P at the neurokinin-1 receptor in the brainstem emetic center and gastrointestinal tract. This is a different mechanism of action than the commonly used serotonin receptor antagonists (ie, ondansetron) for PONV. Another advantage is that Aprepitant is the first long-acting (up to 48 hours) neurokinin-1 receptor antagonist approved for postoperative nausea and vomiting prevention. This medication is significantly more expensive than most other antiemetics, but because it is given as a one-time dose, the additional cost may be worthwhile. Because all patients in this study had general inhalational anesthetics, the findings may not be applicable to plastic surgery procedures done under deep intravenous sedation or monitored anesthesia care sedation.

K. A. Gutowski, MD

What Patients Look for When Choosing a Plastic Surgeon: An Assessment of Patient Preference by Conjoint Analysis
Waltzman JT, Scholz T, Evans GRD (Univ of California, Irvine, Orange)
Ann Plast Surg 66:643-647, 2011

The knowledge of patient preference is crucial for plastic surgeons to determine optimal marketing strategies. Conjoint analysis is a statistical technique whereby research participants make a series of trade-offs. Analysis of these trade-offs reveals the relative importance of component attributes. This study will evaluate the relative importance of attributes that influence the selection and decision-making process when choosing a plastic surgeon. A questionnaire consisting of 18 plastic surgeon profiles was rated by 111 patients. Attributes analyzed were as follows: travel distance, number of years in practice, board certification status, method of referral, office décor, and procedure cost. A traditional full-profile conjoint analysis was performed. Subjects consisted of 10 men and 101 women (n = 111). Median age was 51 years (range, 19–72). The "mean importance" of the attributes are as follows: board certification status, 39.7%; method of referral, 23.5%; distance from home to office, 13.2%; office décor, 9.0%; number of years in practice, 7.5%; and cost of procedure, 7.2%. Internal validity checks showed a high correlation (Pearson $\rho = 0.995$; $P < 0.001$). This pilot study demonstrates that conjoint analysis is a very powerful tool for market research in the health care system. The level of importance for each attribute reliably helps plastic surgeons to understand the preferences of their patients, thus being able to improve marketing strategies for private practices and institutions. The present study indicates that the most important attributes were board certification and method of referral.

► Based on the methodology used and characteristics measured, board certification had the highest "mean importance" for patients choosing a plastic surgeon. This is reassuring and suggests that patients are becoming educated on the importance of board certification. The source of the referral had the second highest mean importance, with a referral from a physician having more utility than a referral from a friend or family member. Other forms of referrals had minimal utility, and surprisingly, the Internet was not rated as being of high utility. However, it could be argued that the Internet and a surgeon's website are powerful entry points into a plastic surgeon's practice, and if a patient never has a chance to enter the practice, he or she will not be able to choose that practice. Furthermore, a "plain and simple" office décor was preferable to a "modern and trendy" or a "traditional and sophisticated" setting. The limitations of this pilot study (based on 4 practices in Southern California with a mix of reconstructive and aesthetic surgery) need to be considered, and hopefully future findings based on larger patient samples with more measurable attributes will be available. However, plastic surgeons should at least consider the evidence we have on patient preferences when designing their practice environment.

K. A. Gutowski, MD

Plastic Surgery Marketing in a Generation of "Tweeting"
Wong WW, Gupta SC (Loma Linda Univ, CA)
Aesthet Surg J 31:972-976, 2011

Background.—"Social media" describes interactive communication through Web-based technologies. It has become an everyday part of modern life, yet there is a lack of research regarding its impact on plastic surgery practice.

Objectives.—The authors evaluate and compare the prevalence of classic marketing methods and social media in plastic surgery.

Methods.—The Web sites of aesthetic surgeons from seven US cities were compared and evaluated for the existence of Facebook, Twitter, or MySpace links and promotions. To find the sites, the authors conducted a Google search for the phrase "plastic surgery" with the name of each city to be studied: Beverly Hills, California; Dallas, Texas; Houston, Texas; Las Vegas, Nevada; Miami, Florida; New York City, New York; and San Francisco, California. The trends of social networking memberships were also studied in each of these cities.

Results.—In comparison to aesthetic surgeons practicing in other cities, those in Miami, Florida, favored social media the most, with 50% promoting a Facebook page and 46% promoting Twitter. Fifty-six percent of New York City aesthetic surgeons promoted their featured articles in magazines and newspapers, whereas 54% of Beverly Hills aesthetic surgeons promoted their television appearances. An increase in the number of new Facebook memberships among cosmetic providers in the seven cities began in October 2008 and reached a peak in October, November, and December 2009, with subsequent stabilization. The increase in the number of new Twitter memberships began in July 2008 and remained at a steady rate of approximately 15 new memberships every three months.

Conclusions.—Social media may seem like a new and unique communication tool, but it is important to preserve professionalism and apply traditional Web site—building ethics and principles to these sites. We can expect continued growth in plastic surgeons' utilization of these networks to enhance their practices and possibly to launch direct marketing campaigns.

▶ Every plastic surgeon encounters patients who are "afraid of needles" and therefore avoid injectable treatments. This non-placebo-controlled trial showed that a simple, commercially available, inexpensive handheld vibration device can decrease the pain associated with Botox injections. This pain reduction modality has been shown to be safe and effective in other situations for pain reduction, most likely by reducing pain transmission from peripheral receptors to the brain. This technique may offer a simple solution for patients who find Botox (and possibly other injections) uncomfortable. Other injection pain reduction strategies include a gentle injection technique, the use of small-gauge needles, prompt replacement of dulled needles, injection of the least possible volume, and topical application of ice packs, cryoanalgesia or vapo-coolant sprays, and anesthetic creams.

K. A. Gutowski, MD

Social Media in Plastic Surgery Practices: Emerging Trends in North America
Wheeler CK, Said H, Prucz R, et al (Univ of Washington, Seattle; et al)
Aesthet Surg J 31:435-441, 2011

Background.—Social media is a common term for web-based applications that offer a way to disseminate information to a targeted audience in real time. In the current market, many businesses are utilizing it to communicate with clients. Although the field of plastic surgery is constantly changing in response to innovative technologies introduced into the specialty, the utilization of social media in plastic surgery practices is currently unclear.

Objectives.—The authors evaluate the current attitudes and practices of aesthetic surgeons to emerging social media technology and compare these to attitudes about more traditional modes of communication.

Methods.—A 19-question web-based survey was disseminated by e-mail to all board-certified or board-eligible American plastic surgeons (n = 4817). Respondents were asked to answer questions on three topics: (1) their use of social media in their personal and professional lives, (2) their various forms of practice marketing, and (3) their demographic information.

Results.—There were 1000 responses (20.8%). Results showed that 28.2% of respondents used social media in their practice, while 46.7% used it in their personal life. Most plastic surgeons managed their social media themselves or through a staff member. The majority of respondents who used social media in their practice claimed that their efforts were directed toward patient referrals. The typical plastic surgery practice that used social media was a solo practice in a large city with a focus on cosmetic surgery. Local competition of plastic surgeons did not correlate with social media use. Most plastic surgeons (88%) advertised, but the form of marketing varied. The most common forms included websites, print, and search engine optimization, but other modalities, such as television, radio, and billboards, were still utilized.

Conclusions.—Social media represents a new avenue that many plastic surgeons are utilizing, although with trepidation. As social media becomes commonplace in society, its role in plastic surgery practice development and communication will become more prominent and defined.

▶ Social media can have a broad definition to include Internet sites such as Facebook (social networking), LinkedIn (professional networking), YouTube (videos), Twitter (brief communications), and blogs (Web-based logs or personal commentaries). They can serve as an adjunct to traditional marketing, particularly with more refined Internet sites, but can also be used on their own to promote a practice. Unlike traditional Internet sites that are more passive and infrequently change content, social media sites are "active" with frequent updates (sometimes daily in the case of Facebook, Twitter, and blogs). Younger and more technology-oriented potential patients are likely to use Facebook as a source of information than more traditional source.

Unlike traditional Internet sites, social media tends to have "followers" who in this case would be established patients or potential patients who came across, or were recommended to, the social media site. So depending on one's practice, social media can be used to inform current (and prospective) patients about new practice events, the surgeon's thoughts on new techniques or products, and comments on plastic surgery—related news. Although it may be a powerful tool to stay in touch with patients, it is not yet a significant source of new patients and referrals for most practices. The patient retention value is more promising. Because this form of marketing requires near daily content and attention, it can require additional resources to incorporate in to a practice. Users also need to be aware of potential legal issues related to patient privacy and Health Insurance Portability and Accountability Act regulation.

K. A. Gutowski, MD

Skin, Soft Tissue, and Hair

Treatment of Axillary Hyperhidrosis With Botulinum Toxin: A Single Surgeon's Experience With 53 Consecutive Patients

Doft MA, Kasten JL, Ascherman JA (Univ Hosps of Cornell and Columbia, NY; Columbia Univ College of Physicians and Surgeons, NY)
Aesthetic Plast Surg 35:1079-1086, 2011

Background.—Axillary hyperhidrosis is a debilitating disease that affects the social and occupational lives of many Americans. It can be treated with subdermal injections of botulinum toxin. This study aimed to determine the interval between injections during which patients are symptom free and whether that interval varies depending on the number of treatments a patient has received.

Methods.—The study enrolled all the patients treated with botulinum toxin for axillary hyperhidrosis by the senior author between 2004 and 2010. Patient responses to the treatment with regard to both satisfaction and length of the symptom-free interval were collected prospectively and analyzed. An in-depth PubMed search was performed through July 2010 to compile the published data on using botulinum toxin injections to treat axillary hyperhidrosis. These data served as a benchmark to which the trends at our institution were compared.

Results.—The 53 patients included in the study had an average age of 29 years, and 64% were women. Of the 53 patients, 23 (43%) underwent multiple injections of botulinum toxin. The average symptom-free interval was 261 days. There was no statistically significant difference in symptom-free intervals after multiple treatments. Patient satisfaction rates were very high, similar to the high degrees of satisfaction found in the published data.

Conclusion.—Botulinum toxin injections provide an effective treatment for axillary hyperhidrosis with a rapid onset and high patient satisfaction. Many patients have a symptom-free interval of 6–9 months after each botulinum toxin injection. This interval does not change significantly after multiple treatments.

▶ For the 1% to 3% of the US population who are affected by significant axillary hyperhidrosis unresponsive to topical treatments, botulinum toxin is a reliable and easy (but somewhat costly) treatment option. Patient evaluation is straight forward, but additional documentation may be needed if insurance coverage is requested. Results typically last 4 to 6 months and may be longer in some patients or for those who have more need during warmer seasons. Although not all patients return for further treatments (typically due to cost), those who do may form a patient base that can then be treated by nurse injectors or other appropriate office staff.

K. A. Gutowski, MD

Treatment of Hyperhidrosis With Botulinum Toxin

Doft MA, Hardy KL, Ascherman JA (Columbia Univ College of Physicians and Surgeons, NY)
Aesthet Surg J 32:238-244, 2012

Botulinum toxin type A is a safe and effective method for treating focal hyperhidrosis, providing longer-lasting results than topical treatments without the necessity of invasive surgical procedures. Although more useful for axillary hyperhidrosis, botulinum toxin injections can also be effective in treating palmar and plantar disease. The effects of botulinum toxin last for six to nine months on average, and treatment is associated with a high satisfaction rate among patients. In this article, the authors discuss their preferred methods for treating axillary, palmar, and plantar hyperhidrosis. This article serves as guide for pretreatment evaluation, injection techniques, and posttreatment care.

▶ For practices that already use Botox (or other similar neuromodulators) for other indications, adding hyperhidrosis treatment is easy and can offer an additional service for patients. The starch iodine test may be used initially, but, in many patients, examining an untreated axilla under loupe magnification will show the extent of sweat production and help determine the area of treatment. While many injection points are needed, they are well tolerated when using a 30-G needle. Treating the palms of the hand and, less commonly, the soles of the feet is harder, as the skin is much more sensitive and thicker, making injections less tolerable. The anesthetic techniques described are reasonable and should be used when treating the hands or feet. Because the cost of botulinum toxins is high, and insurance reimbursement may be low relative to the amount of the product used, a cost analysis should be done before offering this option.

K. A. Gutowski, MD

A Randomized, Blinded Clinical Evaluation of a Novel Microwave Device for Treating Axillary Hyperhidrosis: The Dermatologic Reduction in Underarm Perspiration Study

Glaser DA, Coleman WP, Fan LK, et al (St Louis Univ, MO; Coleman Ctr for Cosmetic Dermatologic Surgery, Metairie, LA; 7/7 Plastic Surgery, San Francisco, CA; et al)
Dermatol Surg 38:185-191, 2012

Background.—Duration of effect and effectiveness limit current options for treating axillary hyperhidrosis. A new microwave procedure for treatment of axillary hyperhidrosis has been tested.

Study Design/Materials and Methods.—Adults with primary axillary hyperhidrosis were enrolled in a randomized, sham-controlled, blinded study. Subjects were required to have a Hyperhidrosis Disease Severity Scale (HDSS) score of 3 or 4 and baseline sweat production greater than 50 mg/5 min. Procedures were administered using a proprietary microwave energy device that isolates and heats target tissue. Responders were defined as subjects reporting a HDSS score of 1 or 2. Subjects were followed for 6 months (sham group) or 12 months (active group).

Results.—Thirty days after treatment, the active group had a responder rate of 89% (72/81), and the sham group had a responder rate of 54% (21/39) ($P < .001$). Treatment efficacy was stable from 3 months (74%) to 12 months (69%), when follow-up ended. Adverse events were generally mild, and all but one resolved over time.

Conclusions.—The procedure demonstrated statistically significant, long-term efficacy in sweat reduction. As with any new procedure, findings from this first investigational device study identified optimization strategies for the future.

▶ The use of botulinum toxin for axillary hyperhidrosis has been incorporated into many plastic surgeons' practices. When patients can no longer tolerate the treatment (due to ineffectiveness or cost), surgical options, most commonly, a sympathectomy, are the next step. A new alternative may be a microwave-based treatment, which causes irreversible thermolysis of apocrine and eccrine glands between the skin and subcutaneous tissue. This microwave device is similar to an office-based laser requiring a large initial investment. Therefore, patient treatment charges are more than for a typical Botox treatment for axillary hyperhidrosis. However, if long-term results are favorable and few or no repeat treatments are needed, this technology may change the primary approach to treating hyperhidrosis.

K. A. Gutowski, MD

Clinical Evaluation of a Microwave Device for Treating Axillary Hyperhidrosis

Hong HC-H, Lupin M, O'Shaughnessy KF (Univ of British Columbia, Vancouver; Miramar Labs, Inc, Sunnyvale, CA)
Dermatol Surg 38:728-735, 2012

Background.—A third-generation microwave-based device has been developed to treat axillary hyperhidrosis by selectively heating the interface between the skin and underlying fat where the sweat glands reside.

Materials and Methods.—Thirty-one (31) adults with primary axillary hyperhidrosis were enrolled. All subjects had one to three procedure sessions over a 6-month period to treat both axillae fully. Efficacy was assessed using the Hyperhidrosis Disease Severity Scale (HDSS), gravimetric weight of sweat, and the Dermatologic Life Quality Index (DLQI), a dermatology-specific quality-of-life scale. Subject safety was assessed at each visit. Subjects were followed for 12 months after all procedure sessions were complete.

Results.—At the 12-month follow-up visit, 90.3% had HDSS scores of 1 or 2, 90.3% had at least a 50% reduction in axillary sweat from baseline, and 85.2% had a reduction of at least 5 points on the DLQI. All subjects experienced transient effects in the treatment area such as swelling, discomfort, and numbness. The most common adverse event (12 subjects) was the presence of altered sensation in the skin of the arm that resolved in all subjects.

Conclusion.—The device tested provided efficacious and durable treatment for axillary hyperhidrosis.

▶ Using the same microwave device as in the above study, long-term improvements in axillary hyperhidrosis were maintained in 90% of patients at 6 and 9 months after treatment, with more than 80% reductions in sweat production from baseline. Although this is a smaller and nonrandomized trial, the results suggest that this new option may be a viable alternative to botulinum toxin for axillary hyperhidrosis.

K. A. Gutowski, MD

Dilution of botulinum toxin A in lidocaine vs. in normal saline for the treatment of primary axillary hyperhidrosis: a double-blind, randomized, comparative preliminary study

Güleç AT (Baskent Univ, Ankara, Turkey)
J Eur Acad Dermatol Venereol 26:314-318, 2012

Background.—Botulinum toxin A (BTX-A) is an effective and safe treatment modality for primary axillary hyperhidrosis. However, some patients experience considerable pain during injections.

Design.—Dilution of botulinum toxin A in lidocaine vs. in normal saline for the treatment of primary axillary hyperhidrosis: a double-blind, randomized, comparative preliminary study.

Objective.—The aim of this study was to compare the efficacy, safety and pain tolerance of lidocaine-diluted BTX-A vs. saline-diluted BTX-A for the treatment of axillary hyperhidrosis.

Methods.—Eight patients were injected with 50 U of BTX-A diluted in 0.5 mL of saline and 1 mL of 2% lidocaine into one axilla and 50 U of BTX-A diluted in 1.5 mL of saline into the other axilla in a randomized fashion. The pain associated with the injections were self-assessed by the subjects using a 100-mm visual analogue scale (VAS).

Results.—Lidocaine-diluted BTX-A and saline-diluted BTX-A were similarly effective regarding the reduction in sweat production, the onset of sweat cessation and the duration of hypo/anhidrosis. Nevertheless, the pain VAS score during the injections was significantly lower in the axilla treated with lidocaine-diluted BTX-A than the one treated with saline-diluted toxin.

Limitations.—Preliminary study due to relatively small sample size.

Conclusion.—Botulinum toxin A diluted in lidocaine causes significantly less pain than BTX-A diluted in saline, whereas it is is equally effective and safe as the latter one in treating axillary hyperhidrosis. Therefore, we suggest that lidocaine-diluted BTX-A may be a better treatment option for the patients with primary axillary hyperhidrosis.

▶ Adding a local anesthetic to botulinum toxin seems to make axillary injection more tolerable. Other techniques include topical anesthetics (which take 30 to 45 minutes to have an effect), skin cooling, and using a 32 G needle. It is unlikely that this technique would be effective for injections to treat palmar or plantar hyperhidrosis. Practitioners should keep in mind that mixing 2 medications together is considered an off-label use.

K. A. Gutowski, MD

A randomized placebo-controlled trial of oxybutynin for the initial treatment of palmar and axillary hyperhidrosis
Wolosker N, de Campos JRM, Kauffman P, et al (Univ of São Paulo Med School and Hosp Albert Einstein, Brazil)
J Vasc Surg 55:1696-1700, 2012

Introduction.—Video-assisted thoracic sympathectomy provides excellent resolution of palmar and axillary hyperhidrosis but is associated with compensatory hyperhidrosis. Low doses of oxybutynin, an anticholinergic medication that competitively antagonizes the muscarinic acetylcholine receptor, can be used to treat palmar hyperhidrosis with fewer side effects.

Objective.—This study evaluated the effectiveness and patient satisfaction of oral oxybutynin at low doses (5 mg twice daily) compared with placebo for treating palmar hyperhidrosis.

Methods.—This was prospective, randomized, and controlled study. From December 2010 to February 2011, 50 consecutive patients with palmar hyperhidrosis were treated with oxybutynin or placebo. Data were collected from 50 patients, but 5 (10.0%) were lost to follow-up. During the first week, patients received 2.5 mg of oxybutynin once daily in the evening. From days 8 to 21, they received 2.5 mg twice daily, and from day 22 to the end of week 6, they received 5 mg twice daily. All patients underwent two evaluations, before and after (6 weeks) the oxybutynin treatment, using a clinical questionnaire and a clinical protocol for quality of life.

Results.—Palmar and axillary hyperhidrosis improved in >70% of the patients, and 47.8% of those presented great improvement. Plantar hyperhidrosis improved in >90% of the patients. Most patients (65.2%) showed improvements in their quality of life. The side effects were minor, with dry mouth being the most frequent (47.8%).

Conclusions.—Treatment of palmar and axillary hyperhidrosis with oxybutynin is a good initial alternative for treatment given that it presents good results and improves quality of life.

▶ Other articles have offered botulinum toxin and microwave energy as treatments for axillary hyperhidrosis. The microwave treatments have not been tested for the less common but perhaps more annoying palmar and plantar hyperhidrosis, and botulinum toxin injections in these areas are difficult because of patient discomfort. Oral oxybutinin (an anticholinergic medication used to relieve urinary and bladder difficulties) may be an alternative for these patients. Thoracic sympathectomy may not be as useful as once thought because of compensatory hyperhidrosis in other areas.

K. A. Gutowski, MD

A Randomized Controlled Trial of Fractional Laser Therapy and Dermabrasion for Scar Resurfacing

Christophel JJ, Elm C, Endrizzi BT, et al (Univ of Virginia Health System, Charlottesville; Boston Univ, MA; Univ of Minnesota, Minneapolis)
Dermatol Surg 38:595-602, 2012

Background.—Dermabrasion has been the standard resurfacing procedure for postsurgical scars, but recovery can be long. Fractionated carbon dioxide (CO_2) laser is a safe, effective tissue resurfacing modality, but no prospective trial has compared its safety or efficacy with that of dermabrasion for postsurgical scar resurfacing.

Objective.—To compare the safety and efficacy of single-treatment fractional photothermolysis with that of single-treatment dermabrasion for postsurgical scar resurfacing on the face.

Methods and Materials.—A split-scar method was used to compare fractionated CO_2 laser and diamond fraise dermabrasion on postsurgical scars of the face. Primary endpoint was safety at day 0, 1 week, and 1 month. Secondary endpoint was efficacy at 3 months as measured by blinded evaluation of standardized photographs.

Results.—Safety data revealed that there was less erythema ($p = .001$) and bleeding ($p = .001$) at day 0, less erythema ($p = .01$) and edema

($p = .046$) at 1 week, and a trend toward less erythema at 1 month ($p = .06$) with fractionated CO_2. Efficacy data at 3 months revealed equivalent scar improvements ($p = .77$).

Conclusion.—Fractionated CO_2 laser therapy should be considered a safe alternative for surgical scar resurfacing on the face. The safety profile exceeds that of dermabrasion, and it has a quicker clinical recovery and equivalent cosmetic efficacy.

▶ Although this small study suggests fractional CO_2 laser treatment may be superior to mechanical dermabrasion for scar treatment, by 3 months the clinical outcomes were similar. Fractional laser technology results in less morbidity and downtime compared to nonfractional laser treatments by creating columns of thermal injury surrounded by noninjured dermal tissue. This allows for faster healing with less complications. Past studies have shown that dermabrasion was better than nonfractionated CO_2 laser treatment for scars, but the newer fractional lasers may now yield better results. Dermabrasion, however, should not be discarded as the devices are less expensive, easier to transport, and have fewer per-use costs than lasers. User experience with both techniques also needs to be considered.

K. A. Gutowski, MD

Investigating the Efficacy of Vibration Anesthesia to Reduce Pain From Cosmetic Botulinum Toxin Injections

Sharma P, Czyz CN, Wulc AE (Drexel Univ College of Medicine, Philadelphia, PA; Ohio Univ College of Osteopathic Medicine, Columbus)
Aesthet Surg J 31:966-971, 2011

Background.—Many analgesic modalities have been employed with limited success to alleviate the pain associated with botulinum toxin type A (BTX-A) injections. Vibration is an effective method of reducing pain during facial cosmetic injections, but it has not been previously studied in the context of clinical cosmetic procedures.

Objectives.—The authors evaluate the safety and efficacy of vibration-assisted anesthesia for reducing pain associated with BTX-A injections.

Methods.—In this prospective study, 50 patients received BTX-A injections for cosmetic rhytid reduction. Injections were given in a split-face design that was randomly assigned. A vibration stimulus was coadministered with BTX-A injections on one side, while the other side of each patient's face received BTX-A injections alone. Patients completed a questionnaire immediately posttreatment and were contacted for follow-up three to four weeks later.

Results.—Patients reported less injection pain on the vibration-treated half of the face as compared to the control side (an average of 1.3 vs 2.4 on a five-point scale; $P = .000$). Overall, 86% of patients preferred to receive vibration with their next BTX-A treatment. There was no significant difference between first-time and repeat BTX-A patients in terms of preference for vibration. Five of 50 patients experienced transient side effects perceived to be associated with vibration, including tingling teeth, increased bruising, and headaches. Of the patients who did not request vibration with subsequent BTX-A injections, none cited decreased BTX-A efficacy as the reason for their preference.

Conclusions.—Vibration is a safe and effective means of reducing patient discomfort during BTX-A injections for cosmetic rhytid reduction and may have applications in other cosmetic procedures.

▶ Every plastic surgeon encounters patients who are afraid of needles and, therefore, avoid injectable treatments. This non-placebo-controlled trial showed that a simple, commercially available, inexpensive handheld vibration device can decrease the pain associated with Botox injections. This pain reduction modality has been shown to be safe and effective in other situations for pain reduction, most likely by reducing pain transmission from peripheral receptors to the brain. This technique may offer a simple solution for patients who find Botox (and possibly other injections) uncomfortable. Other injection pain reduction strategies include a gentle injection technique, the use of small-gauge needles, prompt replacement of dulled needles, injection of the least possible volume, and topical application of ice packs, cryoanalgesia or vapocoolant sprays, and anesthetic creams.

K. A. Gutowski, MD

Hyaluronics for Soft-Tissue Augmentation: Practical Considerations and Technical Recommendations
Beer K, Solish N (Palm Beach Esthetic Dermatology and Laser Ctr, West Palm Beach and Jupiter, FL; Duke Univ, Durham, NC)
J Drugs Dermatol 8:1086-1091, 2009

Hyaluronic acid (HA) fillers are long chains of sugar molecules. Depending on various physical properties, such as chain length and cross-linking, they can have different textures and durations. Injections of hyaluronic acids for soft-tissue augmentation is one of the most popular procedures performed in the U.S., Europe, Asia and Canada. With the development of newer HA molecules, it is likely that this trend will continue. Choosing the right HA for a particular patient depends on various factors, including the area to be treated, skin thickness and patients' risk tolerance. Understanding the various molecules, and how they interact, is essential for ensuring optimal patient outcomes.

▶ The demand for soft tissue injectable fillers for facial rejuvenation continues to increase. The various anatomic treatment areas and expanding range of filler options can make choosing the right filler for the right site challenging and confusing. Even among the commonly used hyaluronic acid products, differences in each product's physical properties can be exploited to achieve better results. It is therefore reasonable to be aware of each product's concentration, amount of cross-linking, shear modulus (G'), and other qualities when deciding on which product to use in a specific anatomic site. For example, the thicker hyaluronic acids are better for deeper creases (such as marionette lines), but thinner products should be used for fine lines (such as upper lip lines). The recommendations in this article include specific product choice for each anatomic treatment site and should be reviewed by surgeons wishing to expand their use of hyaluronic acid fillers.

K. A. Gutowski, MD

An overview of current biomaterials in aesthetic soft tissue augmentation
Ryssel H, Germann G, Koellensperger E (BG-Trauma Centre Ludwigshafen, Germany)
Eur J Plast Surg 35:121-133, 2012

Today an increasing number of patients seek aesthetic improvement through minimally invasive procedures, and interest in soft tissue augmentation and filling agents is rising steadily. However, a thorough understanding of these substances, their indications and contraindications, as well as a profound knowledge of different implantation techniques is essential to provide an aesthetically pleasing result for the patient. This presentation gives an overview of the current injectable biomaterials, their major indications, advantages and disadvantages, with focus on collagen, hyaluronic acid, poly-L-lactide, and autologous fat grafting.

▶ For those beginning to use injectable soft tissue fillers, this overview is worthwhile to better understand the differences between products and identify the ideal indications for use. Even among the commonly used hyaluronic acids, differences in their physical properties can impact the results in certain anatomic regions. Although it is not practical to incorporate every approved filler into one's practice, 1 product for fine lines, 1 for deeper folds, and 1 for overall facial volumization should be available to treat the commonly requested improvements. As more experience is gained, additional products can be added, particularly more long-lasting and semipermanent options.

K. A. Gutowski, MD

Temporal Rejuvenation with Fillers: Global Faceculpture Approach
Raspaldo H (Facial Plastic Surgery Centre, Cannes, France)
Dermatol Surg 38:261-265, 2012

Background.—Nonsurgical temporal rejuvenation techniques are being used increasingly to meet patient demand, but no standardized way for performing them yet exists. Temporal lifts are of most benefit to persons in their mid-30s to early 40s who are beginning to have signs of aging around their eyes. Temporal lifting addresses the sad, tired look without major surgery, lifting the brows, reducing crow's feet lines, firming the outer eye area, and lightening the hooding of the outer eyelid. This approach produces minimal to no scarring, little bleeding, and no hair loss. It is a short procedure with minimal recovery time that can be done in outpatient settings or under twilight anesthesia. The latter entails a 12- to 24-hour hospitalization and a 7- to 15-day recovery period. A review of the pertinent anatomy and products used in temporal rejuvenation was offered, along with recommendations for a nonsurgical approach.

Anatomy and Products.—The temporal area is above the zygomatic arch, between the temporal crest or linea temporalis above and the hairline laterally. Three fascial layers are found, including the superficial temporal fascia, which is strongly attached to subcutaneous tissues, and the superficial and deep layers of the deep temporal fascia, which are attached to the bony floor. The Merkel space, a natural sliding space, is located between the superficial and deep temporal fascial layers. Sensory innervation of the temporal area is supplied by the trigeminal nerve.

Products used in rejuvenation procedures include fillers such as hyaluronic acid (HA), calcium hydroxyl-apatite, poly-L-lactic acid, and botulinum toxin type-A (BoNTA). Cross-linked HA dermal fillers are easy to use and well-tolerated, containing lidocaine to reduce injection pain. Use of an ona-BoNTA and HA combination permits the BoNTA to reduce the activity and volume of the masseter muscles so the temporal muscle has more activity and increases in volume.

Recommended Approaches.—A temporal aging scale can be used at baseline to help guide the choice of esthetic product and determine the volume required before treatment begins. The suggested four stages are 1, normal, convex, or straight temporal fossa; 2, early signs of slight depression; 3, concave temporal fossa and some visible temporal vessels and eyebrow tail droop; and 4, skeletonization of the temporal fossa, with bones visible, veins and arteries obvious, and severe concavity of the fossa. The approaches recommended for each stage are as follows: stage 1, no treatment; stage 2, 0.4 to 0.8 mL of HA filler per side or 0.5 to 1 mL of a volume-restoring product per side; stage 3, 1 to 2 mL of a volume-restoring product per side; and stage 4, 2 to 4 mL of a volume-restoring product per side.

A 27 G needle is recommended with a bolus injection technique to avoid the pain associated with use of a microcannula longer than a needle. A pattern of four sections is physically drawn onto the patient to guide the injections and improve safety. These sections are the zygomatic arch; the lateral part of the orbit, including the curved anterior limit; the linea temporalis fusion zone between the frontal, parietal, and temporal bones, including the curved superior limit; and the hairline. A vertical line is then drawn at the halfway point of the zygomatic arch and a horizontal line from the lateral canthus across. The first injection is designed to refill the anteroinferior quadrant and is the safest and most effective injection point. The needle must penetrate to a depth of 1 to 1.5 cm. If this injection is insufficient, a second injection is performed at the junction of the linea temporalis and superior orbital rim. After this injection is completed, a third injection can be done into the posteroinferior quadrant at the most lateral section of the zygomatic arch. With severe depression an injection can be made into the posterosuperior area. All injections are made as deeply as possible and positioned under the deep temporalis fascia to give more volume projection and avoid the facial nerve. Risks associated with this nonsurgical approach include bruising and pin-prick bleeding, especially when superficial subcutaneous injections are used. Some patients experience mild pain for 1 day and when chewing or biting for 3 to 5 days.

Conclusions.—Nonsurgical temporal rejuvenation is being used more often in response to patient requests. Often it is preferred because there is a short recovery time and the results can be dramatic. An effective approach is to stage the patient at baseline, choose the optimum product and volume needed to obtain the desired result, and then perform injections into the appropriate areas.

▶ Loss of volume in the temporal area is not a common patient complaint, but when severe, the deformity is obvious and contributes to the overall image of an aging face. For many patients, adjusting their hairstyles may cover up the temporal wasting, but with shorter or thinning hair, the deformity becomes more obvious. A prominent zygomatic arch draws even more attention to the temporal hollowness. The use of injectable soft tissue fillers can improve the loss of temporal volume. Just by softening the transition of the bony prominence lateral to the zygoma and superior to the zygomatic arch, a more youthful appearance can be achieved. The technique described uses hyaluronic acid fillers but other longer lasting products (Sculptra or Artefill) may also be used.

K. A. Gutowski, MD

Eyelid

Use of Eye Shields and Eye Lubricants Among Oculoplastic and Mohs Surgeons: A Survey

Ogle CA, Godwin JA, Shim EK (Univ of Southern California, Los Angeles, CA)
J Drugs Dermatol 8:855-860, 2009

Background.—Eye shields and lubricants are recommended for use in the eye during periorbital surgery to prevent injury to the globe. Nonetheless, data regarding their use is sparse, and no study to date has examined the prevalence of their usage and complications.

Purpose.—To investigate how commonly eye shields and lubricants are used during periorbital surgery and whether there are complications from their use.

Methods.—The authors conducted a survey of oculoplastic and Mohs surgery fellowship directors. The questionnaire investigated the prevalence of use of eye shields and lubricants, complications encountered, and whether the standard of care requires or prohibits their use.

Results.—A majority of those surveyed at least sometimes use eye shields in periorbital surgery, particularly to prevent patient injury. Most surgeons believe there are more pros than cons to their use. However, corneal abrasions may be encountered and may be related to the type of lubricant chosen. Surgeons using fat-based lubricants tended to encounter more complications with eye shield use.

Conclusion.—Eye shield and lubricant use is common among oculoplastic and Mohs surgeons. However, most disagree as to whether the standard of care requires or forbids their use.

▶ This survey brings out the fact that despite their ubiquitous use in operating rooms, eye protection methods (shield, tape, and lubricants) do not have a standardized role or logical method of product selection. However, this article is worth reading to become more familiar with the protective options available and the advantages and disadvantages of each, including use in laser cases. At a minimum, surgeons who perform periorbital procedures should be aware of both common complications (corneal abrasion, vision changes, infections, corneal edema) and the rare but potentially devastating injuries (globe perforation) that can occur.

K. A. Gutowski, MD

Face, Neck and Brow

The Safety of Rhytidectomy in the Elderly
Martén E, Langevin C-J, Kaswan S, et al (Cleveland Clinic, OH; M D Anderson Cancer Ctr Orlando, FL; Univ of Rochester, NY)
Plast Reconstr Surg 127:2455-2463, 2011

Background.—The purpose of this study was to evaluate the safety of face-lift surgery in an elderly population. Specifically, is chronologic age an independent risk factor leading to a higher complication rate in the elderly patient undergoing rhytidectomy surgery?

Methods.—The authors retrospectively reviewed consecutive face lifts (216 patients) performed by a single surgeon over a 3-year period. Patients were divided into two groups, younger than 65 years (148 patients) and 65 years and older (68 patients). Comorbidities, operative details, and complications were compared using statistical analysis.

Results.—The average age was 70.0 years in the elderly group and 57.6 years in the younger group. When compared with the patients younger than 65 years, elderly patients were more likely to have a higher American Society of Anesthesiologists score and to have had a prior face lift (41.2 percent versus 17.6 percent, $p < 0.001$). The elderly had complication rates comparable to those of younger patients (2.9 percent versus 2.0 percent major, $p = 0.65$; and 5.9 percent versus 6.1 percent minor, $p = 0.99$). There were no deaths in either group.

Conclusions.—In the authors' series of carefully selected elderly patients, face-lift complication rates were not statistically different when compared with those of a younger control group. The authors' data suggest that chronologic age alone was not an independent risk factor for face-lift surgery.

Further studies are needed to define whether a chronologic age limit for safe face-lift surgery beyond age 65 exists.

▶ Long-term surgical improvement of prominent nasolabial folds is challenging. The anatomy of the region contributes to the progressive formation of the deformity. Lateral to the nasolabial fold, a fat layer surrounds the mimetic muscles and extends superficially to the dermis. A nasolabial fat compartment lies anterior to the medial cheek fat and overlaps the jowl fat. Medial to the nasolabial, there is minimal subcutaneous fat between the dermis and the orbicularis oris muscle where the skin adheres to the muscle directly.

The malar fat pad descends inferiorly and medially with aging. Combined with resorption of the bony malar eminence, this fat pad descent results in a loss of malar prominence and a deeper nasolabial fold. Increased cheek fat volume may contribute to deepening of the fold also. Because the nasolabial fold is made up of dense fibrous tissue and insertions of muscle fibers, the fold will deepen during contraction of the underlying mimetic muscles.

The technique described attempts to address the anatomic contributions to the nasolabial fold by decreasing the bulge lateral to the fold and by dividing the muscle attachments to the dermis. The before and after photos do show improvement of the lateral and inferior nasolabial folds, suggesting that this technique may be useful as a stand-alone procedure or as an adjunct to a facelift.

K. A. Gutowski, MD

Face Lift
Warren RJ, Aston SJ, Mendelson BC (Univ of British Columbia, Canada; New York Univ School of Medicine)
Plast Reconstr Surg 128:747e-764e, 2011

Learning Objectives.—After reading this article, the participant should be able to: 1. Identify and describe the anatomy of and changes to the aging face, including changes in bone mass and structure and changes to the skin, tissue, and muscles. 2. Assess each individual's unique anatomy before embarking on face-lift surgery and incorporate various surgical techniques, including fat grafting and other corrective procedures in addition to shifting existing fat to a higher position on the face, into discussions with patients. 3. Identify risk factors and potential complications in prospective patients. 4. Describe the benefits and risks of various techniques.

Summary.—The ability to surgically rejuvenate the aging face has progressed in parallel with plastic surgeons' understanding of facial anatomy. In turn, a more clear explanation now exists for the visible changes seen in the aging face. This article and its associated video content review the current understanding of facial anatomy as it relates to facial aging. The standard face-lift techniques are explained and their various features, both good and bad, are reviewed. The objective is for surgeons to make a better aesthetic diagnosis before embarking on face-lift surgery, and to have the ability to use the appropriate technique depending on the clinical situation.

▶ The article provides an excellent review of current facelift techniques and new concepts in facial aging that need to be considered when offering a modern facelift procedure. The evolution of thinking about fat compartments, fat redistribution, volume replacement, and attention to retaining ligaments needs to be appreciated. Although there may be no one correct facelift procedure, the various approaches can be used to optimize results for individual patients. The video supplements to this article further expand the written material.

K. A. Gutowski, MD

Long-Term Results of Face Lift Surgery: Patient Photographs Compared with Patient Satisfaction Ratings
Liu TS, Owsley JQ (Aesthetic Surgery Inst, San Francisco, CA)
Plast Reconstr Surg 129:253-262, 2012

Background.—Surgical facial rejuvenation (face lift) remains the aesthetic standard for correction of the anatomical changes of the aging face and for long-lasting results. However, younger patients (younger than 50 years) with early facial aging are often fearful of or discouraged from face-lift surgery in favor of simpler yet short-lived nonsurgical and surgical options. The superficial musculoaponeurotic system—platysma face lift is associated with a high degree of patient satisfaction at 1 year (97.8 percent) and at 12.6 years (68.5 percent). When the satisfaction scores were subdivided into three age groups (younger than 50, 50 to 60, and older than 60 years), the authors found greater satisfaction among the younger age group at the early and long-term intervals. To illustrate these observations, the authors analyzed the photographic results of their survey patients and compared them with their survey results.

Methods.—The photographic results of the patients from our Owsley Facelift Satisfaction Survey were analyzed and stratified into the three age groups. Six patients (two per age group) were included for analysis and are presented for review.

Results.—Patient-rated survey results show that the younger age group consistently scored higher positive ratings, longer lasting aesthetic improvement of their five main anatomical areas of correction, and greater overall satisfaction at long-term follow-up.

Conclusions.—Younger patients with early or minimal signs of facial aging should be considered candidates for surgical facial rejuvenation ("maintenance face lifts") and are the preferred candidates. This age group of patients has consistently positive overall satisfaction with longer lasting facial aesthetic correction.

Clinical Question/Level of Evidence.—Therapeutic, III.

▶ Offering a surgical facelift to younger patients is not easy, given the nonsurgical and minimally invasive options available. Financial concerns, desires for short recovery, and a reluctance to undergo surgery have shifted many patients to injectable facial rejuvenation, which offers favorable results in selected patients. Although this study supports full surgical rejuvenation in patients with early or minimal signs of facial aging, the reality of current patient expectations and economic considerations may make this a tough sell. By the senior author's own admission, he does not "perform or recommend nonsurgical facial aesthetic improvements such as botulinum neuromodulators, injectable dermal fillers, lasers, and chemical peels to his patients." In most practices, the full range of options needs to be available to maintain a viable patient base.

K. A. Gutowski, MD

Cervicofacial Rhytidoplasty: More Does Not Mean Better

Cárdenas-Camarena L, Encinas-Brambila J, Guerrero MT (Centro Médico Puerta de Hierro, Zapopan, Jalisco, Mexico; Mexican Society of Otorhinolaryngology and Head and Neck Surgery, Mexico)
Aesthetic Plast Surg 35:650-656, 2011

Background.—Aesthetic correction of cervicofacial flaccidity has undergone numerous modifications over time, including extent and depth of dissection. We present our experience with this type of surgery, passing through different stages and procedures to achieve optimal and highly satisfactory results.

Methods.—From January 1995 to December 2009, 576 patients (498 females and 78 males, age range = 34—78 years, mean = 47) underwent cervicofacial rhytidoplasty. During the first 6 years of the study period, cervicofacial tissue was managed with six different types of plications, according to the needs of each patient, requiring extensive supra-SMAS undermining. During the last 9 years, undermining was significantly limited and only three of the six plications were used, adding different surgical procedures to achieve the surgical objectives.

Results.—During the first period, 220 patients were operated on and 164 patients required additional procedures (74%). Seventy-nine patients (36%) needed 6 plications, 90 patients (41%) required 5 plications, and 51 patients (23%) only 4 plications. During the second period, 356 patients were operated on, needing only 3 plications, but 336 (94%) required additional procedures. The percentage of complications during the first period was 2.2% hematomas, 2.7% superficial necrosis, and 0.45% deep necrosis compared with 0.84, 0.56, and 0%, respectively, in the second period. A greater disability rate than expected from edema and/or prolonged ecchymosis occurred in 25 and 12% of the patients in the first and second periods, respectively. A similar degree of patient satisfaction was obtained in both periods, 93 and 92%, respectively.

Conclusion.—Our approach to cervicofacial rhytidoplasty has varied substantially by limiting undermining, which has produced a lower complication rate and has accelerated the recovery process. However, to acquire similar results, we have had to implement additional procedures, with which we have obtained the same degree of satisfaction but with a lower rate of postsurgical morbidity.

▶ The SMAS plication technique of the authors appears to give acceptable results, and their evolution to less undermining and less plication maintained patient satisfaction and shortened the recovery period while decreasing the incidence of hematomas and skin necrosis. The initial method involved SMAS plication at the anterior and posterior platysma, malar area, zygomatic arch, midcheek, and preauricular area. After incorporating less undermining, the SMAS was only plicated at the last 3 areas, but anterior neck liposuction was added if needed. Their conclusions of "more does not mean better" supports other less-extensive face lift techniques, especially for younger patients or those with less advanced signs of facial aging. The challenge remains in those patients with significant anterior neck deformities in which limited lateral undermining may not provide lasting results and often leads to higher revision rates. Unfortunately, the authors did not provide information on which patients may have benefited from opening the anterior neck to plicate the platysma.

K. A. Gutowski, MD

Avoiding Complications With Aptos Sutures

Sulamanidze M, Sulamanidze G, Vozdvizhensky I, et al (Plastic Surgeons in private practice, Moscow, Russia; Third Administration of the Russian Federation Health Ministry, Moscow; et al)
Aesthet Surg J 31:863-873, 2011

Background.—Over the past decade, several methods of minimally-invasive thread-mediated lifting have been widely adopted in aesthetic surgery. Early use of these methods met with great enthusiasm, and threadlifting was often performed without sufficient regard for proper indications, controls, or outcomes. Soon after, reports of early-relapse ptosis, complications, and other undesirable side effects began to appear in the literature.

Objectives.—The authors describe the current best practices associated with threadlifting to ensure proper use and improved results.

Methods.—The authors retrospectively reviewed their collective case data, analyzing the results of 12,788 face and neck threadlift procedures in 6098 patients over 12.5 years.

Results.—The data showed inconsistent results and early relapse of deformity with the Aptos Thread and Aptos Thread 2G methods. Complications included thread visibility, migration, and exposure; linear bleeding along the needle course; skin dimpling; hypocorrection and hypercorrection; transient paresthesias; and a small number of cases of injury to major vessels, nerve branches, and parotid capsule/duct. As new devices were developed and the indications for each technique refined, soft tissue suspension became more effective and durable, and the incidence of complications correspondingly decreased in the latter part of the series.

Conclusions.—Threadlifting is a relatively modern trend in aesthetic surgery that demands a similarly novel approach from surgeons. When performed properly, threadlifting is associated with minor and infrequent complications and is a helpful clinical alternative to traditional facial rejuvenation techniques.

▶ Using barbed sutures for facial rejuvenation is much less popular than 5 years ago, perhaps because the results were judged to be short-lasting. This largest series reported to date focuses on the Aptos suture system and offers recommendations for those wishing to use them for facial "threadlifting." The authors acknowledge that initial overuse and poor patient selection and expectations accounted for some of the criticisms of this procedure. They describe their refined protocols based on a newer generation of Aptos sutures and offer advice from their own experience.

Specifically, patient assessment and indications, more detailed techniques, and specific suture selection are offered for each anatomic area. New users of Aptos can decrease complications by:

- Using the suture for the proper indications
- Not placing long threads through 2 or more facial zones
- Paying attention to surgical technique (barb misalignment, injury to vessels or nerves)
- Minimizing over- or undercorrection
- Not placing the Aptos Needle or Aptos Needle 2 G too superficially
- Not using inferior-quality sutures
- Avoiding insertion of tough threads in facial regions where strong muscular activity will work against them.

Despite the decreased popularity of barbed sutures among plastic surgeons in the United States, there may be a role for their use in younger patients who wish to avoid more invasive procedures, need only modest improvements, and are willing to have shorter-lasting results.

K. A. Gutowski, MD

The Percutaneous Trampoline Platysmaplasty: Technique and Experience With 105 Consecutive Patients
Mueller GP, Leaf N, Aston SJ, et al (Private Practice, West Hollywood, CA; UCLA School of Medicine; New York Univ School of Medicine; et al)
Aesthet Surg J 32:11-24, 2012

Background.—Controversy persists regarding the optimal procedure to rejuvenate the aging neck. More invasive procedures carry increased risks of complications, whereas less invasive approaches may deliver marginal results. The challenge is selecting the appropriate procedure for delivering consistent, durable results meeting both the patient's and surgeon's expectations.

Objectives.—The authors describe their trampoline platysmaplasty (TPP) approach, a percutaneous suture suspension necklift that constitutes a less invasive approach for neck rejuvenation.

Methods.—A retrospective study was conducted of 105 consecutive patients who underwent TPP. Age, sex, procedure(s) performed, complications, and patient satisfaction were recorded. Cadaver studies were conducted to compare the tensile strength of the ligaments that anchor the TPP to the tensile strength of the sutures placed to approximate the medial platysma borders. In addition, the accuracy of light transillumination to determine depth of travel of the light-emitting diode (LED) lighted rod was evaluated.

Results.—Patients underwent either TPP alone (18 women, 24 men) or TPP with a facelift (35 women, 28 men) between October 2007 and June 2009. The average age of the patients was 52 years, and average length of follow-up was 33 months. Patient satisfaction was high. Three early patients underwent immediate revision to improve results secondary to the suture matrix being too loose. Six additional patients had recurrent banding around one year postoperatively, but correction was achieved in all six by replacing the matrix with the help of the lighted rod. The results of the cadaver study revealed that the tensile strength of the retaining ligaments was statistically identical to the medial platysma borders, and the light transillumination feedback was accurate with regard to the depth of travel of the illuminated rod tip.

Conclusions.—The TPP approach for neck rejuvenation is effective and durable in properly-selected patients. It works well as a stand-alone procedure and in conjunction with facelift procedures. It also offers younger patients a less-invasive option to improve neck contours inherited through genetics. After nearly three years of follow-up of the patients in this report, the results appear to be long-lasting (Fig 14).

▶ The percutaneous suture suspension trampoline platysmaplasty (TPP) described in this article was done using the iGuide Surgical Suture System, which was invented by the lead author. The technique requires a specialized light-guided system to percutaneously place sutures around the mandibular, retaining ligaments in a "shoelace" pattern to provide improved submental and neckline contour. Patient selection was appropriately considered as those who had only submental fat deposition that could be treated with liposuction alone were excluded. Likewise, patients with large necks and excessive redundant neck skin were treated with traditional open techniques and were not included either. Since some of the patients underwent a concurrent facelift, it is hard to measure the degree of neck improvement related to TPP versus the facelift. However, in the cases where the TPP was used alone or with liposuction, favorable results are seen (Fig 14). This technique may be a good option for younger

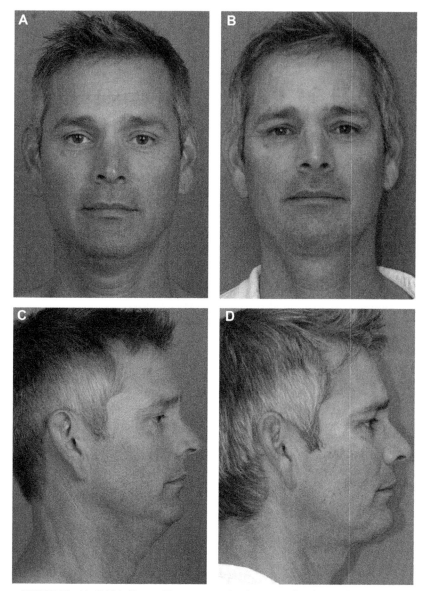

FIGURE 14.—(A, C) This 42-year-old man presented with a genetically-inherited obtuse cervicomental angle and ptotic submandibular glands. (B, D) Thirty-one months after undergoing neck liposuction and trampoline platysmaplasty. (Reprinted from Mueller GP, Leaf N, Aston SJ, et al. The percutaneous trampoline platysmaplasty: technique and experience with 105 consecutive patients. *Aesthet Surg J.* 2012;32:11-24, with permission from The American Society for Aesthetic Plastic Surgery, Inc.)

patients with milder neck deformities who are seeking a less-invasive procedure. After some experience, it should be possible to perform this procedure using local anesthetic.

K. A. Gutowski, MD

The Minimal Access Deep Plane Extended Vertical Facelift
Jacono AA, Parikh SS (North Shore Univ Hosp, Manhasset, NY; Plastic Surgeon in Private Practice in Cupertino, CA)
Aesthet Surg J 31:874-890, 2011

Background.—Modern facelift techniques have benefited from a "repopularization" of shorter incisions, limited skin elevation, and more limited dissection of the superficial musculoaponeurotic system (SMAS) and platysma in order to shorten postoperative recovery times and reduce surgical risks for patients.

Objectives.—The authors describe their minimal access deep plane extended (MADE) vertical vector facelift, which is a hybrid technique combining the optimal features of the deep plane facelift and the short scar, minimal access cranial suspension (MACS) lift.

Methods.—The authors retrospectively reviewed the case records of 181 patients who underwent facelift procedures performed by the senior author (AAJ) during a two year period between March 2008 and March 2010. Of those patients, 153 underwent facelifting with the MADE vertical technique. With this technique, deep plane dissection releases the zygomaticocutaneous ligaments, allowing for more significant vertical motion of the midface and jawline during suspension. Extended platysmal dissection was utilized with a lateral platysmal myotomy, which is not traditionally included in a deep plane facelift. The lateral platysmal myotomy allowed for separation of the vertical vector of suspension in the midface and jawline from the superolateral vector of suspension that is required for neck rejuvenation, obviating the need for additional anterior platysmal surgery.

Results.—The average age of the patients was 57.8 years. The average length of follow-up was 12.7 months. In 69 consecutive patients from this series, average vertical skin excision measured 3.02 cm on each side of the face at the junction of the pre auricular and temporal hair tuft incision (resulting in a total excision of 6.04 cm of skin). Data from the entire series revealed a revision rate of 3.9%, a hematoma rate of 1.9%, and a temporary facial nerve injury rate of 1.3%.

Conclusions.—The common goal of all facelifting procedures is to provide a long-lasting, natural, balanced, rejuvenated aesthetic result with few complications and minimal downtime. The MADE vertical facelift fulfills these criteria and often yields superior results in the midface and neck areas, where many short scar techniques fail. Furthermore, this procedure can be performed under local anesthesia, which is a benefit to both patients and surgeons.

▶ This facelift technique is a fusion of the MACS (minimal access cranial suspension) lift and a more traditional "deep plane" (superficial musculoaponeurotic system (SMAS) and skin elevation) lift. There are data that support better longevity and fewer revisions for a deep plane lift compared with a lateral SMASectomy, and so incorporating a deep plane component to a MACS lift may offer an advantage for a better long-term result. In these authors' practice, a large number of their minimal access deep plane extended facelifts were done to correct prior lateral SMASectomy procedures or MACS lifts that had early recurrent jowls or neck deformities. This more invasive MACS lift variant has a steeper learning curve because the deep plane elevation is more complex than with other SMAS procedures. The published results are satisfactory, and patient selection should focus on the ideal patients who do not have significant neck deformities.

K. A. Gutowski, MD

Vertical Subperiosteal Mid-face-lift for Treatment of Malar Festoons
Hoenig JF, Knutti D, de La Fuente A (Univ Hosp and Med School of Goettingen, Germany)
Aesthetic Plast Surg 35:522-529, 2011

Background.—Malar mounds may be accentuated by chronic lid edema, with the development from malar edema to malar mounds and finally to malar festoons. Because standard techniques do not seem effective and not specifically proposed for the treatment of malar festoons, subperiosteal vertical upper-midface lift associated with lower blepharoplasty overcomes these shortcomings.

Methods.—Twelve patients (3 males and 9 females, age = 47 ± 6 years) underwent video-assisted endoscopic subperiosteal vertical upper-midface lift (SUM-lift) in conjunction with a lower blepharoplasty between 2006 and 2007 for treatment of malar festoons. This includes simultaneous lower blepharoplasties and video-assisted transtemporal subperiosteal and sub-SMAS tissue release.

Results.—All patients healed uneventfully without any major postoperative problems. The surgical outcome was evaluated according to the analysis of photographs obtained before and after surgery and the analysis of pre- and postoperative measurements. The technique we used (SUM-lift) achieved a significant rejuvenation of the midface and the malar festoons.

Conclusion.—Subperiosteal vertical midface lift resuspends and redrapes the facial network that originates at the level of the orbital rim. It seems to improve the permeability characteristics of the malar septum in the treatment of malar festoons and malar mounds by freeing the cheek tissue

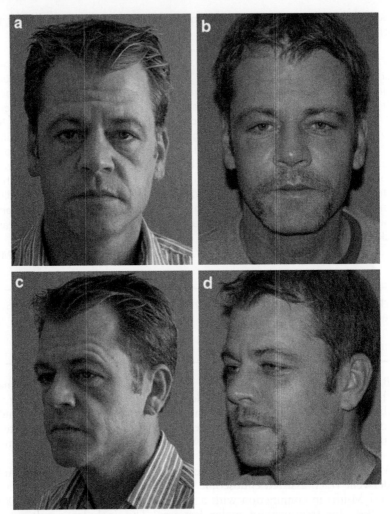

FIGURE 14.—a, c Preoperative views of a 48-year-old patient. He demonstrates ptosis of the malar tissues, loose festoons, hollowing of the infraorbital area, lengthening of the lower eyelid, attendant tear-trough deformity, and nasojugal grooves. b, d Six months after a vertical upper-midface lift (SUM-lift) the nasojugal groove is reduced, the length of the lower lid is shortened, the festoon is removed, and the eyelid-cheek junction is enhanced to a more youthful position with increased malar projection. (Reprinted from Hoenig JF, Knutti D, de la Fuente A. Vertical subperiosteal mid-face-lift for treatment of malar festoons. *Aesthetic Plast Surg.* 2011;35:522-529, with kind permission from Springer Science+ Business Media.)

from underlying bone and redraping the malar septum. It is a reliable technique to improve malar mounds, palpebral bags, or festoons (Fig 14).

▶ Malar mounds and festoons are much more challenging to treat than simple lower eyelid fullness due to fat herniation. This approach gives nice results (seen in Fig 14) and demonstrates the power of a midface lift with adequate soft tissue release and redraping. The video-assisted component of this technique can probably be omitted, as much of the dissection can be achieved with an intraoral incision and lower lid incision.

K. A. Gutowski, MD

Surgical Softening of the Nasolabial Folds by Liposuction and Severing of the Cutaneous Insertions of the Mimetic Muscles
Wang J, Huang J (Southern Med Univ, People's Republic of China)
Aesth Plast Surg 35:553-557, 2011

Background.—A surgical technique was developed to soften the nasolabial folds by liposuction and severing of the cutaneous insertions of the mimetic muscles. This procedure was used for 11 patients from September 2006 to June 2009.

Methods.—With the patients under local tumescent anesthesia, extraoral incisions were made in nine cases and intraoral incisions in two cases. Liposuction was performed superior and lateral to the nasolabial fold using an order-made one-hole 2.5-mm cannula. After liposuction, the fibrae septa and the cutaneous insertions of the mimetic muscles in the nasolabial region were severed by a sharp-edge eye scissors. Compressive dressings were maintained for 3 days.

Results.—All the patients, followed up from 3 months to 3 years, were satisfied with the aesthetic results. Both the depth and the length of the nasolabial folds were decreased conspicuously. The most obvious change was improvement in the lateral part of the nasolabial folds. The extraoral scars were almost imperceptible. Severe complications were not observed in this series.

Conclusion.—Surgical softening of the nasolabial folds by liposuction and severing of the cutaneous insertions of the mimetic muscles is especially suitable for 40- to 60-year-old women with aging faces who are unwilling to undergo a face-lift. The procedure is simple, and the anatomic causes for deepening of the nasolabial folds can be corrected. Patients usually are satisfied with the final postoperative results.

▶ Long-term surgical improvement of prominent nasolabial folds is challenging. The anatomy of the region contributes to the progressive formation of the deformity. Lateral to the nasolabial fold, a fat layer surrounds the mimetic muscles and extends superficially to the dermis. A nasolabial fat compartment lies anterior to the medial cheek fat and overlaps the jowl fat. Medial to the nasolabial, there is minimal subcutaneous fat between the dermis and the orbicularis oris muscle where the skin adheres to the muscle directly.

The malar fat pad descends inferiorly and medially with aging. Combined with resorption of the bony malar eminence, this fat pad descent results in a loss of malar prominence and a deeper nasolabial fold. Increased cheek fat volume may contribute to deepening of the fold also. Because the nasolabial fold is made up of dense fibrous tissue and insertions of muscle fibers, the fold will deepen during contraction of the underlying mimetic muscles.

The technique described attempts to address the anatomic contributions to the nasolabial fold by decreasing the bulge lateral to the fold and by dividing the muscle attachments to the dermis. The before and after photos do show improvement of the lateral and inferior nasolabial folds, suggesting that this technique may be useful as a stand-alone procedure or as an adjunct to a facelift.

K. A. Gutowski, MD

Open Neck Lipectomy for Patients With HIV-Related Cervical Lipohypertrophy
Ion L, Raveendran SS (Chelsea and Westminster Hosp, London, UK)
Aesthetic Plast Surg 35:953-959, 2011

Background.—The advent of effective antiviral medications has revolutionised the management of the HIV-infected patients. Although this has helped in achieving prolonged symptom control, high numbers of these patients are left with the stigmata of complications associated with the medication. Lipodystrophy, either as lipoatrophy or lipohypertrophy, is a known complication of long-term HIV infection and aggressive antiviral therapy, leading to significant physical and psychological morbidity in these patients.

Methods.—Eleven patients demonstrating HIV-related anterolateral neck lipohypertrophy were offered the option of an open cervicoplasty involving pre- and subplatysma lipectomy, platysmaplasty, liposuction, and face-lift in selected patients.

Results.—The amount of adipose tissue excised from each patient was higher than that normally achieved through liposuction, with the highest total of 140 g in one patient. The degree of cervical contouring was significant, with all patients reporting profound satisfaction in terms of restoration of a cosmetically acceptable neck contour. Complications included two hematomas and one seroma. There was no incidence of infection.

Conclusion.—Open anterior cervicoplasty with subplatysma contouring is a powerful tool for predictable and safe results and should be considered as one of the valuable treatment options for HIV-related anterolateral neck lipohypertrophy. Although the incidence of complications is higher than that for similar non-HIV patients, the degree of improvement it provided was perceived by patients as very rewarding.

▶ Cervical lipohypertrophy in human immunodeficiency virus patients with highly active antiretroviral therapy is commonly treated with liposuction. In cases where the fatty deposits are subplatysmal, liposuction is not an option, and an open technique for fat excision is required. This is a much more aggressive approach, and the extended subplatysmal dissection and tissue excision may result in a higher risk for nerve injuries. The results, however, are much more dramatic than with liposuction alone. An initial CT or MRI study may be useful in determining the extent of subplatysmal fat that will need to be addressed.

K. A. Gutowski, MD

Liposuction for highly active antiretroviral therapy (HAART)-associated lipohypertrophy
Malahias M, Lemonas P, Ghorbanian S, et al (Barts and the London NHS Trust, Whitechapel, UK, et al)
Eur J Plast Surg 35:5-8, 2012

The aim is to explore satisfaction levels in HIV patients following liposuction for HAART-associated lipodystrophy. Ninety postal questionnaires were sent out, enquiring about regions affected and scoring the improvement in lifestyle, discomfort and time of recurrence. We received 66 replies (73%). All areas showed significant patient satisfaction and improvement of lifestyle as well as decrease in the discomfort previously experienced. The area with the marginally lower score was the abdomen while the interscapular and occipital area that comprised the majority of patients with the same complaint was found to have high scores of satisfaction from the patients treated. Liposuction is beneficial in managing antiretroviral-associated lipohypertrophy. Patients should be warned of variable recurrence rates and satisfaction outcomes for each anatomical region addressed.

▶ Correction of lipohypertrophy in human immunodeficiency virus patients with highly active antiretroviral therapy can have unpredictable results. The tissue deformity tends to be more fibrous and therefore more difficult to remove. There also seems to be a higher recurrence rate, and subsequent treatments in the same regions are even less likely to yield a significant improvement. Despite these challenges, patients may report a high satisfaction rate, particularly in the "buffalo hump" area, since the deformities tend to be significant and interfere with activities. Patients should be advised about the 20% to 30% recurrence rate, which can happen in less than 6 months.

K. A. Gutowski, MD

Combination Laser-Assisted Liposuction and Minimally Invasive Skin Tightening with Temperature Feedback for Treatment of the Submentum and Neck
Alexiades-Armenakas M (Yale Univ, New Haven, CT)
Dermatol Surg 38:871-881, 2012

Background.—There is need for better nonsurgical treatment of excessive neck fat and skin laxity.

Objective.—To assess combination laser-assisted liposuction (LAL) and minimally invasive skin tightening (MIST) of the submentum and neck under direct temperature control.

Design.—Randomized, prospective, three-arm study of single LAL-MIST treatment comparing 1,064, 1,319 nm, and blended 1,064 and 1,319 nm.

Methods.—Twelve subjects were randomized to three arms. LAL was fiber administered into the adipose layer, followed by aspiration. MIST was laser fiber administered into the subdermal plane. Multiple passes were administered until uniform 45−48°C was attained in the targeted plane. Energy delivery totalled 5,000−7,000 J. Subjects were photographed at baseline and 1, 2, 3, 4, 5, and 6 months after treatment and assessed using a 4-point quantitative laxity grading scale and fat aspirate quantitation.

Results.—Mean ± standard deviation baseline, follow-up, and difference in laxity grades and percentage improvement over baseline for the three study arms and total were 3.19 ± 0.38%, 1.88 ± 0.85%, 1.31 ± 0.55%, and 43.8 ± 18.5%, respectively, for 1,064 nm; 3.75 ± 0.29%, 2.38 ± 0.25%, 1.38 ± 0.25%, and 36.6 ± 5.9%, respectively, for 1,319 nm; 3.38 ± 0.48%, 2.13 ± 0.63%, 1.25 ± 0.29%, and 39.3 ± 12.9%, respectively, for 1,064/1,319 nm; and 3.44 ± 0.43%, 2.13 ± 0.61%, 1.31 ± 0.36%, and 39.4 ± 12.1%, respectively, total. Mean fat aspirate volumes were 6.13 ± 3.28 mL for 1,064 nm, 8.25 ± 2.50 mL for 1,319 nm, and 6.50 ± 5.74 mL for 1,064/1,319 nm. Clinical improvement was consistent across all subjects; all before-and-after photographs are presented (save a recognizable subject for privacy). No blistering, scarring, or dyspigmentation was observed.

Conclusion.—Combination temperature-controlled LAL-MIST treats excess fat and skin laxity of the submentum and neck with excellent safety and efficacy.

▶ External and internal energy treatments (focused ultrasound scan, radiofrequency, and lasers) are being promoted for skin tightening in the face and body. The energy delivered stimulates collagen production by increasing the tissue temperature, resulting in skin contraction. The extent of skin tightening is difficult to quantify objectively, but a few recent studies found statistically significant improvements with internal laser techniques combined with liposuction. Despite the statistical improvement, the level of clinical improvement is modest at best compared with nonlaser-assisted liposuction. The minimally invasive skin tightening technique delivers energy directly into the dermis or subdermal plane through needle electrodes or fiber optic cannulas. As with the other energy delivery devices, internal or external tissue temperature monitoring is needed to prevent skin burns. This pilot study found that similar levels of improvement were seen in all 3 laser wavelengths used. However, a control group of just liposuction without laser was not included. Based on a critical review of all the before and after images in this series, the results are similar (and no better) than what would be expected after traditional nonlaser-assisted liposuction. As with most other noninvasive options, this is not an alternative to a properly performed surgical face or neck lift.

K. A. Gutowski, MD

Lipofilling With Minimal Access Cranial Suspension Lifting for Enhanced Rejuvenation

Willemsen JCN, Mulder KM, Stevens HPJD (Plastic Surgeons in Private Practice in The Hague, Netherlands)
Aesthet Surg J 31:759-769, 2011

Background.—Loss of volume is an important aspect in facial aging, but its relevance is frequently neglected during treatment.

Objectives.—The authors discuss lipofilling as an ancillary procedure to improve the impact of facelifting procedures.

Methods.—Fifty patients who underwent minimal access cranial suspension (MACS) lifting alone were retrospectively analyzed, and their results were compared to 42 retrospective cases of MACS lifting with adjuvant lipofilling. The results were evaluated with a photographic ranking system by two panels (five plastic surgeons and five medical students).

Results.—Combined MACS lifting and lipofilling yielded overall cosmetic results that were significantly better than the results achieved with MACS lifting alone. Photographic evaluations showed that improvements were more pronounced in the tear trough ($P < .05$) and malar eminence ($P < .01$) than in the nasolabial groove ($P > .05$).

Conclusions.—Volume restoration with lipofilling following MACS lifting procedures produces significantly better postoperative results than MACS lifting alone. This combined procedure produces the most dramatic improvements in the tear trough and malar eminence regions.

▶ The minimal access cranial suspension lift has become popular as a less-invasive facelift option for mild to moderate facial aging. As with most facelift techniques, it does not restore volume but rather elevates the superficial muscu-loaponeurotic system, offering some deep tissue repositioning. Using structural fat grafting in the central face, particularly the infraorbital area, can offer a more balanced result by reversing volume loss. Likewise, fat injections to the nasola-bial folds and deeper perioral creases are an excellent addition to most facelift techniques that typically do not address these problem areas.

K. A. Gutowski, MD

Intranasal Surgical Approach for Malar Alloplastic Augmentation

de la Peña-Salcedo JA, Soto-Miranda MA, Lopez-Salguero JF (Inst for Plastic Surgery, Mexico City, MX)

Aesthet Surg J 32:27-38, 2012

Background.—Alloplastic malar augmentation is becoming an increasingly common procedure for enhancement of the midface and an adjunct method of improving the effects of other rejuvenation procedures.

Objectives.—The authors present a new surgical approach for placement of malar implants by means of an intranasal incision, which they believe has several advantages over traditional techniques. They also propose a new classification for regions of the midface to assist in augmentation planning.

Methods.—Between 1990 and 2010, the authors treated 20 patients with an intranasal approach for alloplastic malar augmentation. Patients were preoperatively divided into three groups: Type 1 included those with adequate nostril opening, including good elasticity of the internal nasal mucosa, allowing a good exposure of the piriform aperture through the nasal speculum; Type 2a included those with inadequate nostril opening; and Type 2b included those who required an alar base correction. Implants were selected according to these classifications and placed with the authors' technique.

Results.—Of the 20 patients treated, 18 were female and two were male. Ages ranged from 15 to 65 years. Average follow-up was 10 years, and all patients experienced favorable results. There were no major complications, no nerve or vascular supply compromise, and no cases of implant malposition. One patient requested removal of the implant at one year postoperatively despite her good postoperative outcome; overall patient satisfaction was 95%.

Conclusions.—The intranasal approach for alloplastic malar augmentation has shown good results for midface enhancement in the authors' hands. In this patient series, results showed excellent overall patient satisfaction and a very low (nearly 0%) complication rate.

▶ The 5 approaches for malar augmentation are intraoral (perhaps the most common), transpalpebral, transconjunctival, transcoronal, and through a rhytidectomy incision. The authors found the intranasal approach to be significantly easier than the intraoral approach. Potential advantages over the intraoral approach include less risk of inferior displacement because the pocket dissection is completely horizontal, which helps to maintain a sturdy ledge upon which the implant can rest. Avoiding the intraoral approach may also decrease the risk of infection. However, this technique will work only for soft silicone implants because the porous implants may be too rigid to pass through the smaller incision.

K. A. Gutowski, MD

Nose

A New Method That Uses Cyanoacrylate Tissue Adhesive to Fill Scoring Incisions in Septal Cartilage Correction

Özyazgan İ, İdacı O (Erciyes Univ, Kayseri, Turkey)
Laryngoscope 121:1164-1172, 2011

Objectives/Hypothesis.—Numerous methods are used in the correction of deviated septal cartilage. One of these methods is to perform partial-thickness incisions (scoring) on the concave side of the deviated cartilage. In this retrospective report, we present a series of patients who were treated by filling the scoring incision gaps with cyanoacrylate-based tissue adhesives to increase the effectiveness of scoring incisions and to maintain stability of the corrected concave cartilage segments.

Study Design.—A retrospective clinical study presenting a patient group who was treated using a new surgical method for septal deviation.

Methods.—Twenty-three patients with septum deviation and nasal deformity underwent surgery with the open rhinoplasty approach. Intra- or extracorporeal scoring incisions were performed on the concave side of the deviated septal cartilage, and cyanoacrylate tissue adhesives were applied to the incisions of the corrected cartilage. After polymerization and hardening of the cyanoacrylate tissue adhesive, the operation continued in the normal manner. Preoperative and postoperative clinical results and computed tomography images of the patients were assessed.

Results.—With a mean 24-month follow-up, all patients with respiratory complaints related to deviated septum reported improvement in nose breathing. Clinical and radiologic observations showed that the corrected septum was stable in its new position. There were no complications arising from the use of cyanoacrylate.

Conclusions.—Cyanoacrylate is an effective, instant, safe method of treatment in correcting deviated septal cartilage with scoring incisions and filling the gaps of the incisions (Fig 4).

▶ One of the most difficult aspects of dealing with the "crooked nose" in my experience is correcting the septal deviation and maintaining that correction

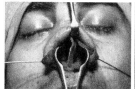 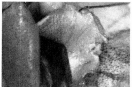 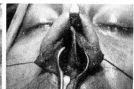

FIGURE 4.—*Left*, deviated septal cartilage; *middle*, intracorporeal scoring incisions made on the concave side of the cartilage in different directions; *right*, overcorrected septal cartilage after CA application to scoring incisions. [Color figure can be viewed in the online issue, which is available at wileyonlinelibrary.com.] (Reprinted from Özyazgan İ, İdacı O. A new method that uses cyanoacrylate tissue adhesive to fill scoring incisions in septal cartilage correction. *Laryngoscope.* 2011;121:1164-1172, with permission from The American Laryngological, Rhinological and Otological Society, Inc.)

over time. Scoring, degree and depth, and the use of cartilage/bone or nonbiological materials have not universally proven to be successful for the immediate result and, more important, in many reports documenting long-term evaluations. This report details the benefits of using cyanoacrylates (CAs) to fill the gaps created when scoring the septal cartilage to correct and maintain the deviation, a technique that appears promising (Fig 4 composite). Especially intriguing is the statement that the use of CAs may reduce the difficulties that result from scoring too deeply or not deeply enough. Study and use of this technique by other surgeons to confirm these results would be helpful in assessing its place in the armamentarium of nasal surgeons.

S. H. Miller, MD

Outcomes research in rhinoplasty: Body image and quality of life
Cingi C, Songu M, Bal C (Eskisehir Osmangazi Univ Med Faculty, Turkey; Izmir Ataturk Res and Training Hosp, Izmir, Turkey)
Am J Rhinol Allergy 25:263-267, 2011

Background.—Although hundreds of quality-of-life (QOL) studies are available in the literature, very few were designed that include both a global and a procedure-specific evaluation of QOL and an inventory for the assessment of body image. The purpose of this study was to use condition-specific and global measures as well as psychological evaluations in a case series of rhinoplasties for a more comprehensive assessment of patient-reported outcomes.

Methods.—Records of 225 patients aged 18—57 years who underwent rhinoplasty were prospectively included in the study. Study participants completed both a baseline questionnaire before the rhinoplasty operation and a postsurgical patient questionnaire 12 months after the operation, including the European QOL Questionnaire (EQ), Rhinoplasty Outcomes Evaluation Questionnaire (ROE), and the Multidimensional Body—Self Relations Questionnaire (MBSRQ).

Results.—Mean values corresponding to the EQ VAS results except for discomfort and anxiety domains increased after treatment compared with baseline. Both male and female patients experienced significant improvement in ROE scores, with larger differences between pre- and postoperative ROE scores in male patients compared with female patients. The analyses of variance in the MBSRQ results revealed significant postsurgical improvements on the appearance orientation subscale.

Conclusion.—The development, standardization, and use of validated procedure-specific QOL tools are essential components for accurately measuring patient-reported outcomes of facial plastic surgery procedures. To measure patient satisfaction in a more objective and standardized manner, specific questionnaires or instruments should be used that can determine the QOL changes associated with each procedure of interest.

▶ Outcomes research in aesthetic plastic surgery has, for the most part, been rare. The authors have performed such a study using several types of quality of life (QOL) tools, including the European generic QOL tool, a multidimensional body-self relations tool and a tool that specifically relates to changes in patients' subjective evaluation following rhinoplasty. The study considered 225 patients between the ages of 18 and 57 and did distinguish between gender but did not look into differences in postoperative perceptions based on age differences; these subjective results also were not correlated with any objective findings. One wonders why the authors chose not to use the Derriford Appearance Scale,[1] a well-studied, valid, and reliable scale for the assessment of difficulty living with cosmetic deformity.

S. H. Miller, MD

Reference

1. Carr T, Harris D, James C. The Derriford Appearance Scale (DAS-59): a new scale to measure individual responses of living with problems of appearance. *Br J Health Psychol.* 2000;5:201-215.

Creeping anaesthesia for nasal surgery—a relatively painless technique
Pandya AN, Harb A, Bayne DR (The Royal Hosp Haslar, Hampshire, UK)
Eur J Plast Surg 34:457-458, 2011

Enzymatically charged local anaesthesia was induced in 42 patients undergoing soft tissue nasal tip, lateral nasal wall, alar and perinasal surgery. This was achieved by means of a standard local anaesthetic combined with hyaluronidase injected in the region of the root of the nose. Complete nasal anaesthesia was achieved in all patients within 60 sec of the local anaesthetic being deposited. No further local anaesthetic infiltration was required at any other site on the nose. This technique ensured a relative degree of comfort to the patient during the administration of the local anaesthetic and furthermore prevented any anaesthetic water logging of the tissues.

▶ This is an interesting article, albeit, of an old idea often published in the ophthalmologic literature and used for peribulbar anesthesia.[1] It has also been cited in otology and laryngology literature regarding anesthesia for nasal fracture manipulation.[2] However, it does not seem to have made its way into the plastic surgery literature for use as an adjunct to local anesthesia for nasal surgery. It certainly seems as if hyaluronidase would be worthwhile for use in cosmetic surgery under local anesthesia requiring multiple injections of the local anesthetic. Combined with preinjection EMLA it might even render the entire local anesthetic experience painless.

S. H. Miller, MD

References

1. Nathan N, Benrhaiem M, Lotfi H, et al. The role of hyaluronidase on lidocaine and bupivacaine pharmacokinetics after peribulbar blockade. *Anesth Analg.* 1996;82:1060-1064.
2. Clement WA, Vyas SH, Marshall JN, Dempster JH. The use of hyaluronidase in nasal infiltration: prospective randomized controlled pilot study. *J Laryngol Otol.* 2003;117:614-618.

Can Elimination of Epinephrine in Rhinoplasty Reduce the Side Effects: Introduction of a New Technique

Kalantar-Hormozi A, Fadaee-Naeeni A, Solaimanpour S, et al (Shahid Beheshti Med Univ, Tehran, Iran; Guilan Univ of Med Sciences, Iran; Persian General Hosp, Tehran, Iran; et al)
Aesthetic Plast Surg 35:582-587, 2011

Background.—We aim to provide evidence that despite not administering epinephrine, (1) the amount of hemorrhaging during surgery will not change, (2) surgery time will not increase and may even be shorter, and (3) there would be fewer cardiovascular-related consequences.

Methods.—One hundred thirteen patients were enrolled and randomized into the control ($n = 74$) and intervention groups ($n = 39$). During the primary open or closed rhinoplasty operation, anesthesia was managed by continual infusion of remifentanil (14–20 µg/h) and propofol (4–6 mg/kg/h) with an infusion pump, in addition to N_2O-O_2 (50%). Atracurium was repeated (5 mg every 20 min). Patients in the control group received an epinephrine (1/100,000) injection to the nose, and patients in the intervention group did not. All patients received dexamethasone (8 mg IV) and metoclopramide (10 mg IV). At the end of the operation and before extubation, the muscle relaxants were reversed with prostigmine (0.35 mg/kg) and atropine (0.175 mg/kg).

Results.—We found (1) no statistically significant association between epinephrine injection and hemorrhage during or after surgery ($P = 0.949$), (2) a statistically significant association between epinephrine injection and complications, and (3) the group that did not receive the injection had fewer complications ($P = 0.01$). With respect to the duration of surgery, we did not detect any statistically significant associations between the groups.

Conclusion.—Elimination of epinephrine during rhinoplasty as an alternative procedure may lead to the same surgery outcomes if not a better one. Studies with a larger sample size are needed to further substantiate these findings.

▶ This is an interesting study, the results of which must be viewed carefully for several reasons. Although it was randomized to a degree, care was taken to ensure that those needing septoplasty were equally divided between treatment and nontreatment groups. Furthermore, patients in the study group did not receive epinephrine, or any injection, during the course of the procedure. One could ask why the patients in the control group, those not receiving epinephrine/ lidocaine, did not receive saline injections so as to "blind" the surgeons perform-ing the procedures? One also wonders why the authors chose not to use cocaine for preparation in their patients and why they chose 1:100 000 as the preferred concentration of epinephrine. We have found, and reported, that the use of 5% cocaine during rhinoplasty is relatively safe and epinephrine in concentrations of 1:400 000 was locally effective when injected in a wide variety of tissues without causing significant systemic symptoms.[1,2] Nonetheless, the suggestions made by the authors are valuable to consider, and further study is certainly war-ranted by those choosing to use general anesthesia for rhinoplasty. Of course, the results of this study may not be relevant for those choosing to use local anes-thesia plus sedation during the performance of rhinoplasty/septoplasty.

S. H. Miller, MD

References

1. Miller SH, Buck DC, Woodward WR, Demuth RJ. Alterations in local blood flow and tissue-gas tension caused by epinephrine. *Plast Reconstr Surg.* 1984;73: 797-803.
2. Miller SH, Dvorchik B, Davis TS. Cocaine concentrations in the blood during rhinoplasty. *Plast Reconstr Surg.* 1977;60:566-571.

Extremity and Trunk

Surgical Correction of Gynecomastia in Thin Patients

Cigna E, Tarallo M, Fino P, et al (Univ of Rome, Italy)
Aesthetic Plast Surg 35:439-445, 2011

Background.—Gynecomastia refers to a benign enlargement of the male breast. This article describes the authors' method of using power-assisted liposuction and gland removal through a subareolar incision for thin patients.

Methods.—Power-assisted liposuction is performed for removal of fatty breast tissue in the chest area to allow skin retraction. The subareolar incision is used to remove glandular tissue from a male subject considered to be within a normal weight range but who has bilateral grade 1 or 2 gynecomastia.

Results.—Gynecomastia correction was successfully performed for all the patients. The average volume of aspirated fat breast was 100—200 ml on each side. Each breast had 5—80 g of breast tissue removed. At the 3-month, 6-month, and 1-year follow-up assessments, all the treated patients were satisfied with their aesthetic results.

Conclusions.—Liposuction has the advantages of reducing the fat tissue where necessary to allow skin retraction and of reducing the traces left by surgery. The combination of surgical excision and power-assisted lipo-plasty also is a valid choice for the treatment of thin patients.

▶ Liposuction is a useful adjunct when excising gynecomastia, even in thin patients. It allows for easier excision of the glandular tissue due to creation of tunnels in the subcutaneous space. It also results in smoothing of the contour irregularities after excision of the glandular tissue. Because the fatty tissue in the chest may be more fibrous than in other regions, power-assisted or ultrasound-assisted liposuction makes the procedure easier compared with traditional liposuction. Using a power-assisted arthroscopic-endoscopic cartilage shaver may allow for complete fibrous tissue excision without a periareolar incision. The authors compare the outcomes and complications of their results to other similar techniques; however, the sample size is too small to draw conclusions about which technique is best.

K. A. Gutowski, MD

Venous Thromboembolism in Abdominoplasty: A Comprehensive Approach to Lower Procedural Risk
Somogyi RB, Ahmad J, Shih JG, et al (Univ of Toronto, Ontario, Canada)
Aesthet Surg J 32:322-329, 2012

Background.—Venous thromboembolism (VTE) is a serious and potentially life-threatening surgical complication. However, there is little consensus regarding appropriate VTE prophylaxis for plastic surgery patients. Risk factors as they apply to plastic surgery patients are unclear, and recent recommendations for chemoprophylaxis in these patients may expose them to other additional risks.

Objectives.—The authors examine perioperative and intraoperative measures, specifically those that have enabled a large number of patients to undergo outpatient abdominoplasty safely, with a reduced risk of VTE.

Methods.—A retrospective review was performed of 404 consecutive abdominoplasty patients who were treated at a single outpatient surgery center between 2000 and 2010. Graded compression stockings and intermittent pneumatic compression devices were placed on all patients, and perioperative and intraoperative warming was strictly applied. Progressive tension suturing technique was performed in all cases and drains were eliminated. All patients received pain pumps, ambulated within one hour of surgery, and were discharged home the same day. Patient VTE risk factors were scored with the Caprini/Davison risk assessment model (RAM). Perioperative and intraoperative measures were taken to reduce factors that may increase VTE risk in abdominoplasty. Complications were recorded, including VTE events, seromas, hematomas, and infections.

Results.—In this series, 247 abdominoplasty procedures were performed alone and 157 were combined with additional procedures. Under the RAM, 297 patients were considered "high risk" and 17 "highest risk." Abdominoplasty operative time was 100 ± 29 minutes. Only one case of deep vein thrombosis (DVT) occurred, in the calf.

Conclusions.—A comprehensive approach to perioperative and intraoperative patient care has allowed outpatient abdominoplasty to be safely performed without VTE chemoprophylaxis in patients with fewer than six risk factors.

▶ Abdominoplasty, alone or in combination with other procedures, seems to be associated with a higher risk of venous thromboembolism (VTE) than other aesthetic procedures. Despite the increased risk, there is resistance to providing chemoprophylaxis to abdominoplasty patients for fear of bleeding complications. The Caprini recommendations and subsequent American Society of Plastic Surgeons VTE prophylaxis recommendations (http://www.plasticsurgery.org/ Documents/medical-professionals/health-policy/key-issues/VTE_Risk_Assessment_ and_TF_Recommendations.pdf) help stratify patients into graded risk groups, which should allow for a more patient-specific approach to VTE prevention. The strategy described in this article is reasonable because it promotes early ambulation, maintenance of normothermia, and use of lower extremity intermittent compression devices. Although abdominoplasty-specific VTE prophylaxis recommendations do not yet exist, based on results of other plastic surgery procedures, chemoprophylaxis should be strongly considered for the highest-risk patients.

K. A. Gutowski, MD

Abdominoplasty with Suction Undermining and Plication of the Superficial Fascia without Drains: A Report of 113 Consecutive Patients

Rodby KA, Stepniak J, Eisenhut N, et al (Florida State Univ and Lentz Plastic Surgery, Daytona Beach)
Plast Reconstr Surg 128:973-981, 2011

Background.—Postoperative abdominoplasty seromas are a problem. Although drains are still commonly used during the initial postoperative period, this article has demonstrated that the combination of an extended incision, suction undermining, and progressive tension sutures can produce superior results without the need for suction drains.

Methods.—A retrospective review of 113 consecutive abdominoplasty patients operated on between April of 2004 and May of 2010 was carried out and complications were reviewed.

Results.—There were 109 women and four men, with ages spanning 23 to 76 years (average, 50 years). Complications of the surgery included hematoma (2.7 percent), with one requiring drain placement (0.9 percent) and two treated with needle aspiration (1.8 percent); seroma (8.8 percent), with four requiring closed suction drainage (3.5 percent) and six minimally treated with needle aspiration (5.3 percent); infection (2.7 percent), with one requiring intravenous antibiotics (0.9 percent) and two with minimal local erythema (1.8 percent); and minimal marginal skin necrosis with spontaneous healing (3.5 percent).

Conclusions.—The technique of abdominoplasty with the addition of an extended incision, liposuction undermining of the deep fatty tissue between the superficial and abdominal muscle fascia, and the use of progressive tension sutures results in a better abdominal wall and waist contour. This decreases the need for dissection of the abdominal panniculus above the umbilicus except for a small tunnel to allow for the suturing of the rectus abdominis muscles. This allows for preservation of the arterial and lymphatic vessels, improving blood flow to the superior flap and decreasing seroma formation to the point where operative drains are not required.

Clinical Question/Level of Evidence.—Therapeutic, IV.

▶ This report suggests that the subcutaneous tissue below the umbilicus is not needed to preserve lymphatic flow after abdominoplasty as a technique to prevent seroma formation. Also, the tissue from the incision to the umbilicus can be excised down to the abdominal wall fascia without leaving a layer of deep fat. As others have demonstrated, progressive tension sutures allow for elimination of drains in abdominoplasty and lipoabdominoplasty.

K. A. Gutowski, MD

Intraoperative Assessment of the Umbilicopubic Distance: A Reliable Anatomic Landmark for Transposition of the Umbilicus
Rodriguez-Feliz JR, Makhijani S, Przybyla A, et al (Albany Med Ctr, NY; et al)
Aesthetic Plast Surg 36:8-17, 2012

Background.—A clear understanding of the anatomic location and the aesthetic traits of the umbilicus is essential for the plastic surgeon repositioning the umbilicus during an abdominoplasty. Currently no consensus exists regarding the ideal location for this unique aesthetic unit of the abdomen. To their interest, the authors noted that the intraoperative distance from the pubic symphysis to midumbilical stalk measured 15 cm for several consecutive patients. They believe the umbilicopubic distance is another clinically useful and reliable anatomic landmark for the plastic surgeon relocating the umbilicus during an abdominoplasty.

Methods.—A retrospective chart review analysis was performed for 40 consecutive patients who underwent abdominoplasty or panniculectomy between July 2009 and May 2010 at the authors' institution. The intraoperative measurement of the umbilicopubic distance (pubic symphysis to midumbilical stalk) was available for 32 of these patients. The average umbilicopubic distance was calculated. Two separate graphs were generated to evaluate the relationship of the umbilicopubic distance to the patients' height and body mass index (BMI). The data were saved and analyzed using Microsoft Office Excel.

Results.—In the study population, the average intraoperative umbilicopubic distance was found to be 15.05 cm. The results validate the mean umbilicopubic distance of 15.04 cm reported by Dubou and colleagues in 1978. For patients whose stature fell between 145 and 178 cm, the umbilicopubic distance was consistently 15 cm. A tendency toward a higher umbilicus was noted as the patients became taller. The BMI did not seem to influence the location of the umbilicus as measured intraoperatively.

Conclusion.—Translocation of the umbilicus to 15 cm from the pubic symphysis in patients with a stature of 145–178 cm is another clinically useful, safe, and expeditious method for relocation of the umbilicus during an abdominoplasty.

▶ Classic teaching is that the umbilicus is located at the level between the third and fourth lumbar vertebrae (a landmark not very useful during abdominoplasty), at a point 3 cm superior to the anterior superior iliac spine or at the superior level of the iliac crest. In practical terms, during an abdominoplasty, the umbilicus should be positioned at the same level as the patient's own umbilical stalk attachment to the abdominal wall. The opening on the abdominal flap may be placed a bit lower to form a "superior hood," which may be more aesthetically pleasing and helps hide the superior scar. In massive weight loss patients or those with inferior umbilical displacement due to severe skin laxity, the new position of the umbilicus will typically be somewhat more superior and the stalk may need to be shortened before attachment to the abdominal skin. The 15-cm distance should be considered in limited abdominoplasties when the stalk is divided and the umbilicus is pulled inferiorly along with the skin flap. If displaced too low (more than 2 to 3 cm), the abdominal proportions may be disrupted, resulting in a poor aesthetic outcome. Although tall patients with a superiorly set umbilicus may tolerate a 3-cm or more inferior transposition, shorter patients may not.

K. A. Gutowski, MD

Does Abdominoplasty Have a Positive Influence on Quality of Life, Self-Esteem, and Emotional Stability?
Papadopulos NA, Staffler V, Mirceva V, et al (Munich Technical Univ, Germany; Hosp of Dachau, Germany; et al)
Plast Reconstr Surg 129:957e-962e, 2012

Background.—In a previous prospective study, the authors evaluated the quality of life in patients undergoing aesthetic surgery. In this survey, the authors split up the operative indication and analyzed quality of life, self-esteem, and emotional stability after abdominoplasty alone.

Methods.—Sixty-three patients participated in the study. The testing instrument consisted of a self-developed questionnaire to collect demographic and socioeconomic data and a postoperative complication questionnaire developed especially for abdominoplasties. In addition, a standardized self-assessment test on satisfaction and quality of life (Questions on Life Satisfaction), the Rosenberg Self-Esteem Questionnaire, and the Freiburg Personality Inventory were used.

Results.—Significantly increasing values in some items of the standardized self-assessment test on satisfaction and quality of life were found: sum scores of the General Life Satisfaction showed a significant improvement ($p = 0.004$) and the scores of the items housing/living conditions ($p = 0.000$) and family life/children ($p = 0.000$). Within the Satisfaction with Health module, a significant improvement in the items mobility ($p = 0.02$) and independence from assistance ($p = 0.01$) was found. Values in the module Satisfaction with Appearance (Body Image) increased regarding satisfaction with the abdomen ($p = 0.001$). Over 84 percent were very satisfied with the aesthetic result, 93.4 percent would undergo the same treatment again, and 88.9 percent would further recommend the operation. Data revealed that participants' self-esteem was very high and their emotional stability was very well balanced.

Conclusions.—This study demonstrates that abdominoplasty increases most aspects of quality of life, particularly family life, living conditions, mobility, and independency from assistance. Also, patient self-esteem and emotional stability ratings are very high postoperatively.

▶ Most plastic surgeons already know that in properly selected patients, aesthetic body contouring procedures have a high satisfaction rate and generate more referrals. This study may be useful in counseling prospective abdomino-plasty patients who may be unsure about undergoing the procedure by present-ing them the objective data on quality of life and self-esteem improvement.

K. A. Gutowski, MD

Rectus sheath plication in abdominoplasty: Assessment of its longevity and a review of the literature

Tadiparthi S, Shokrollahi K, Doyle GS, et al (Royal Victoria Infirmary, UK; Whiston Hosp, Merseyside, UK; Countess of Chester Hosp, Cheshire, UK)

J Plast Reconstr Aesthet Surg 65:328-332, 2012

Background.—Correction of rectus diastasis during abdominoplasty is controversial. Few published studies have investigated the long-term value of plication. This prospective study aims to assess the long-term dura-bility of plication of the rectus sheath in abdominoplasty using ultrasound.

Methods.—A total of 28 consecutive abdominoplasty patients underwent rectus plication by the senior author (FSF) since 2006, using a 0/0 looped nylon suture. Rectus diastasis was measured preoperatively and postopera-tively at 3, 6 and 12 month's intervals using a standardised ultrasound (7.5 MHz) probe, by the single senior radiologist (GJD). Diastasis of the recti was assessed at three fixed points: at the umbilicus, 6 cm above and 6 cm below the umbilicus. Diastasis was categorised using the Beer classification.

Results.—All patients were female with a mean age of 36 years and average of body mass index (BMI) 26 kg m^{-2}. The majority of subjects had previous abdominal surgery including caesarean sections (82%, $n = 23$) and had at least one previous pregnancy (87%), with only two patients (8.7%) in the study being nulliparous. Correction of diastasis was maintained in all patients despite previous pregnancies and abdominal surgery.

Postoperative follow-up time averaged 28 months (range 12—43 months). According to the Beer classification, there was no recurrence of rectus diastasis at the 12-month postoperative ultrasound measurements. A significant reduction in the mean distance between rectus muscles before surgery and 12 months postoperatively was noted. Previous surgery did not have a statistically significant affect on preoperative rectus distance.

Conclusions.—Vertical rectus plication with a non-absorbable suture demonstrates long-term durable results without any suture-related complications. Patient factors such as extent of preoperative rectus diastases and previous abdominal surgery did not appear to have a significant effect on the durability of the corrected diastasis.

▶ A small percentage of patients seem to lose the benefit of a rectus sheath plication after abdominoplasty. The specific plication technique and suture material used have not been studied extensively, but from the few plastic surgery and general surgery studies, permanent monofilament or long-lasting dissolvable sutures may be better than braided permanent or shorter-acting dissolvable sutures. A single layer continuous vertical plication is common, but a 2-layer plication or an interrupted suture plication may prevent disruption of the repair during the early postoperative period. In addition to the vertical plication, small transverse plications are useful to correct bulges in the midabdomen and around the umbilicus. Patients should be advised that some relapse may occur based on weight changes, intraabdominal fat, muscle tone, and tissue quality.

K. A. Gutowski, MD

"Uro-Abdominoplasty": An Adaptation of Abdominal Contouring for Revision of Complicated Urostomies

Mickute Z, Chen Y-A, Som R, et al (Univ of Cambridge, UK; Addenbrooke's Univ Hosp, Cambridge, UK)
Ann Plast Surg 68:295-299, 2012

Background.—The aim of this study was to describe the indications, surgical technique and outcomes of abdominoplasty as a novel tool for revising complicated urostomies.

Patients and Methods.—Four patients (3 female, 1 male; mean body mass index = 32 kg/m^2; mean age = 56 years) who underwent abdominoplasty for urostomy revision 2007–2009 were identified. Ileal conduits had been performed following ablative or diversion surgery for cervical carcinoma, bladder carcinoma, interstitial cystitis, and neuropathic bladder. A postal questionnaire was used to establish pre- and postabdominoplasty stoma function.

Results.—Patients were referred to the reconstructive team with problems fitting their urostomy-appliance leading to urinary leakage, skin irritation, and social embarrassment. Uro-abdominoplasty indications included multiple abdominal scars (n = 2), large abdominal apron (n = 4), and deep skin creases (n = 2). Three patients had undergone previous failed urostomy repositioning or peristomal liposuction. The joint plastic surgical-urological operations lasted a mean of 3 hours, with no major postoperative complications. Patients were discharged 8 days later. Of 4 patients, 3 reported improved appliance fitting and reduced urinary leakage (>50%) and the remaining patient had intermittent leakage due to a persistent abdominal fold superiorly, and has since undergone reverse abdominoplasty. Two patients complained of long-term lower abdominal numbness, but all 4 were satisfied with the aesthetic improvement.

Conclusions.—Abdominoplasty has been successfully used in our center for the purpose of improving urostomy dysfunction of intractable mechanical leakage by creating a flatter surface for appliance fitting. Uro-abdominoplasty widens the reconstructive repertoire of plastic surgeons and can be considered in those who have exhausted conservative or simpler surgical solutions.

▶ The versatility of plastic surgery allows us to use aesthetic principles and procedures for reconstructive purposes. For patients with urostomy dysfunction due to abdominal wall contour irregularities, an abdominoplasty-like procedure, can improve function and quality of life after other options (stoma revision or relocation) are exhausted. Based on personal experience, liposuction may also be used in selected cases where the problem is limited to a smaller part of the abdominal wall. These principles may also be used for dysfunctional intestinal ostomies.

K. A. Gutowski, MD

Buttock Augmentation With Solid Silicone Implants

Senderoff DM (Plastic Surgeon in Private practice in New York City)
Aesthet Surg J 31:320-327, 2011

Background.—Buttock augmentation with solid silicone implants has become an increasingly popular procedure in the United States, but few outcomes studies have been undertaken to evaluate its safety and efficacy.

Objective.—The author examines the results of buttock augmentation with solid silicone implants in his private practice.

Methods.—A retrospective chart review was conducted of 200 consecutive patients who underwent bilateral buttock augmentation with a total of 400 solid silicone implants over an eight-year period from June 2001 through August 2009. Implants were placed in the subfascial position in 154 patients and in the intramuscular position in 46 patients. Most intramuscular implant placements occurred early in the series, before the author refined his technique. Data from all patients were analyzed to determine the rate of complication, need for surgical revision, and aesthetic outcome.

Results.—Twenty-six men and 174 women were included in the study. The mean duration of follow-up was three years. The overall reoperation rate for these patients was 13% (n = 26). Seroma formation was the most common complication, occurring in 28% (n = 56) of patients. The infection rate was 6.5% for both subfascial and intramuscular implants (n = 13). The implant infection rate was 3.8% (15 of the 400 implants). Hematoma formation occurred in 2% (n = four) of patients. Wound dehiscence occurred in 1.5% (n = three) of patients. Capsular contracture was noted in 1% (n = two) of patients. Data showed that additional aesthetic procedures at the time of buttock augmentation did not affect the complication rate. In terms of patient satisfaction, patients with intramuscular implants complained more often about a lack of inferior gluteal fullness.

Conclusion.—Buttock augmentation with solid silicone implants is a safe and satisfying procedure for both patient and surgeon. The most common complication in this series was seroma formation, which was treated with serial aspiration in most cases. Gluteal implants were successfully placed in either the subfascial or intramuscular position with no significant difference in complication rate, but subfascial implant placement can produce better aesthetic results in patients requiring inferior gluteal fullness.

▶ Most reports of buttock and gluteal implant augmentation are from outside the United Sates and, therefore, may be based on implants that are not available to American plastic surgeons. This series used the solid silicone elastomer implants that are currently available in the United States.

The overall reoperation rate was 13%, which approaches that for breast implants, but the indications for reoperation were different. Overall infection affected 6.5% of patients with 11 of 13 patients requiring implant removal (with 4 subsequent successful replacements done later), and the remaining 2 patients were treated for cellulitis. *Staphylococcus aureus* was cultured in 11 of 13 cases, suggesting that prophylactic antibiotics should be selected based on skin pathogen coverage and that a proper skin preparation is done. Aesthetic indications for reoperation were less common and included 2 patients who desired larger implants, 2 patients who complained of palpability with their subfascial implants, and 2 patients who complained of intramuscular implant displacement.

Based on this author's experience, a few points are worth considering when comparing intramuscular (IM) versus subfascial (SF) gluteal implant placement:

- Patients with IM implants complained more often about a lack of inferior gluteal fullness.
- IM patients required more time to recuperate and complained of more pain than SF patients.
- Final aesthetic results were evident more quickly in SF patients than in IM patients.
- SF implants exhibited better overall buttock projection.

Also, patient selection considerations include:

- The best candidates were women with ample subcutaneous buttock fat and good skin elasticity.
- A short, round buttock was found to be more amenable to round implants than a long buttock, where oval implants were placed on occasion.
- In patients with infragluteal fold skin ptosis after implantation, cresenteric skin excision can be performed.
- Poor candidates for buttock augmentation include obese patients because of difficult dissection and postoperative shearing forces on the implant and

wound. Extremely thin patients with inadequate soft tissue coverage are also poor candidates for buttock implantation.

Given the options of fat grafting versus implant buttock augmentation, the patient's body habitus and tissue qualities should be considered. Each method has advantages and disadvantages that need to be discussed with a potential patient.

K. A. Gutowski, MD

Autologous Gluteal Lipograft

Nicareta B, Pereira LH, Sterodimas A, et al (Policlinca Geral, Rio de Janeiro, Brazil; LH Clinic, Rio de Janeiro, Brazil; et al)

Aesthetic Plast Surg 35:216-224, 2011

In the past 25 years, several different techniques of lipoinjection have been developed. The authors performed a prospective study to evaluate the patient satisfaction and the rate of complications after an autologous gluteal lipograft among 351 patients during January 2002 and January 2008. All the patients included in the study requested gluteal augmentation and were candidates for the procedure. Overall satisfaction with body appearance after gluteal fat augmentation was rated on a scale of 1 (poor), 2 (fair), 3 (good), 4 (very good), and 5 (excellent). The evaluation was made at follow-up times of 12 and 24 months. The total amount of clean adipose tissue transplanted to the buttocks varied from 100 to 900 ml. In nine cases, liponecrosis was treated by aspiration with a large-bore needle connected to a 20-ml syringe, performed as an outpatient procedure. Infection of the grafted area also occurred for four patients and was treated by incision drainage and use of antibiotics. Of the 21 patients who expressed the desire of further gluteal augmentation, 16 had one more session of gluteal fat grafting. The remaining five patients did not have enough donor area and instead received gluteal silicone implants. At 12 months, 70% reported that their appearance after gluteal fat augmentation was "very good" to "excellent," and 23% responded that their appearance was "good." Only 7% of the patients thought their appearance was less than good. At 24 months, 66% reported that their appearance after gluteal fat augmentation was "very good" (36%) to "excellent" (30%), and 27% responded that their appearance was "good." However, 7% of the patients continued to think that their appearance was less than good. At this writing, the average follow-up time for this group of patients has been 4.9 years. The key to successful gluteal fat grafting is familiarity with the technique, knowledge of the gluteal topography, and understanding of the patient's goals. With experience, the surgeon can predict the amount of volume needing to be grafted to produce the desired result. Although the aim of every surgeon is to produce the desired augmentation of the gluteal region by autologous fat grafting in one stage, the patient should be advised that a secondary procedure may be needed to accomplish the desired result.

▶ Buttock augmentation with autologous fat grafting (popularly called the "Brazilian butt lift") typically requires much higher fat graft volumes than other fat-grafting procedures, such as those in the face or breast. This prospective report of 351 patients with 1- and 2-year patient-reported evaluations showed surprisingly high patient satisfaction. Using a syringe aspiration fat harvest method and minimal saline wash syringe separation, the typical total fat graft volume was 200 to 400 mL with only a small portion of patients receiving more than 600 mL.

At 2 years, only 7% of patients considered their appearance as "less than good," and there appeared to be a correlation of the injected fat volume and patient satisfaction. The patients who rated their result as excellent at 2 years had 270 to 740 mL (mean, 575 mL) injected, whereas the patients who rated their result as poor or less than poor had 130 to 290 mL (mean, 190 mL) injected. However, there also seemed to be a correlation between the amount of fat injected and the fat necrosis complication rate.

K. A. Gutowski, MD

Use of dermal fat graft for augmentation of the labia majora

Salgado CJ, Tang JC, Desrosiers AE III (Univ of Miami, FL)
J Plast Reconstr Aesthet Surg 65:267-270, 2012

Dermal fat grafts have been utilized in plastic surgery for both reconstructive and aesthetic purposes of the face, breast, and body. There are multiple reports in the literature on the male phallus augmentation with the use of dermal fat grafts. Few reports describe female genitalia aesthetic surgery, in particular rejuvenation of the labia majora. In this report we describe an indication and use of autologous dermal fat graft for labia majora augmentation in a patient with loss of tone and volume in the labia majora. We found that this procedure is an option for labia majora augmentation and provides a stable result in volume-restoration.

▶ Changes in the female pubic area due to aging or massive weight loss may result in decreased labia majora fullness and increased size of the labia minora. Although rarely a functional problem, the aesthetic changes may be a concern for some women. In addition, there are data that suggest there is enhanced sexual function after labioplasty (typically a reduction of excess tissue) and vaginoplasty for both women and their sexual partners.[1] Cases of injectable poly-L-lactic acid (Sculptra) volumization of the labia majora have been reported, and fat injections may also be used. In cases where excised tissue is available from another procedure being done at the same time (ie, abdominoplasty), a dermal fat graft may be a reasonable option to restore a more youthful and balanced appearance to the vulva. If a labia minora reduction is planned at the same time as a labia majora procedure, the patient should be prepared for more edema in the area than with a labia minora procedure alone.

K. A. Gutowski, MD

Reference

1. Goodman MP, Placik OJ, Benson RH 3rd, et al. A large multicenter outcome study of female genital plastic surgery. *J Sex Med.* 2010;7:1565-1577.

Liposuction

A fifteen-year experience of buttock contouring with combination of silicone implant, liposuction, and structural fat grafting

Karacaoglu E, Durak N (Yeditepe Univ, Istanbul, Turkey)
Eur J Plast Surg 35:81-87, 2012

Buttock augmentation is one of the most popular procedures to shape and augment the gluteal region. The major literature regarding this topic accentuates the role of the implant in gluteal shaping. The goal of this study is to present our personal experience and approach while emphasizing the role of implant positioning and structural fat grafting to yield a more satisfied buttock contouring. Gluteal implants were placed with various orientation mostly the more spherical portion facing inferiorly to simulate the round shape of the midportion of the gluteal region as an alternative to its classical positioning. Patients were analyzed based on the projection as well as the shape and contour of buttocks. Gluteal contouring with rationale positioning of the gluteal implants combined with structural fat grafting may play a role to yield a more satisfied buttock contouring.

▶ Buttock augmentation has gained more popularity in the United States but not yet to the extent as in other countries. The traditional procedure used prosthetic implants, but fat grafting has become more common. This study combined both methods, allowing for more specific areas of augmentation and lower fat injection volumes (70 to 140 cc) and also incorporated liposuction for additional contouring. The implants were gel-filled (not currently available in the United States) and placed in an intramuscular pocket. Although this dissection is a bit more difficult than a subcutaneous or subfascial pocket, it may give a more natural appearance and lower the risk of capsular contracture. The fat grafts were placed in layers (intramuscular, just above the muscle, and subcutaneous) depending on the specific desired effect of augmentation. This combined approach to gluteal contouring may be ideal for correcting asymmetries and enhancing volume in areas where implants typically are less effective, such as the lateral buttock.

K. A. Gutowski, MD

Prospective Outcome Study of 360 Patients Treated with Liposuction, Lipoabdominoplasty, and Abdominoplasty
Swanson E (Private Practice, Leawood, KS)
Plast Reconstr Surg 129:965-978, 2012

Background.—Patient-reported data, including effects on quality of life, have not been previously prospectively evaluated in liposuction patients, or in abdominoplasty patients treated simultaneously with liposuction. This prospective outcome study was undertaken to evaluate and compare liposuction and abdominoplasty from the patient's perspective.

Methods.—From 2002 to 2007, in-person interviews were conducted with 360 patients who attended a follow-up appointment at least 1 month after surgery, from a total of 551 consecutive patients treated with ultrasonic liposuction and/or abdominoplasty (response rate, 65.3 percent). Questions were asked in six categories: patient data, indications, recovery, results, complications, and psychological effects. Responses were analyzed in three groups: liposuction alone ($n = 219$), combined liposuction and abdominoplasty ($n = 128$), and abdominoplasty alone ($n = 13$).

Results.—For most recovery indices, liposuction patients recovered significantly more quickly than lipoabdominoplasty patients ($p < 0.01$) and had less discomfort (pain ratings, 6.1 of 10 and 7.5 of 10, respectively; $p < 0.001$). The result ratings for lipoabdominoplasty (9.0 of 10) and abdominoplasty (8.7 of 10) were higher than for liposuction alone (7.8 of 10; $p < 0.001$). Overall, 85.8 percent of patients reported improved self-esteem and 69.6 percent reported an improved quality of life.

Conclusions.—Liposuction and abdominoplasty, either alone or in combination, provide high levels of patient satisfaction (88.8 percent overall). The combined procedure is similar in discomfort level to abdominoplasty alone (both 7.5 of 10) and produces the highest level of patient satisfaction (99.2 percent), with 97.6 percent of patients saying they would undergo the operation again and 99.2 percent recommending it to others.

Clinical Question/Level of Evidence.—Therapeutic, II.

▶ Although this is a single surgeon's outcomes report, the findings are useful as they can likely be applied to most body contouring practices, perhaps even as a benchmark of what results to strive for in one's own patients. One interesting observation was that approximately half of all patients reported that the amount of liposuction was "not enough." This may be an area where more patient education and emphasis on realistic expectations should be offered. Despite this finding, over 80% of liposuction patients reported that their expectations had been met. Overall, liposuction and abdominoplasty, individually and in combination, have patient satisfaction rates and generally improve self-esteem.

K. A. Gutowski, MD

A Liposuction Technique for Extraction of Bio-Alcamid and Other Permanent Fillers

Khan I, Shokrollahi K, Bisarya K, et al (Morriston Hosp, Swansea, UK)
Aesthet Surg J 31:344-346, 2011

Bio-Alcamid (Polymekon Research, Brindisi, Italy) is a permanent soft tissue filler that has been injected for the correction of contour deformities. It has a number of indications, including pectus excavatum. Infection and migration seem to be the most common complications with this product. The authors report an illustrative case of pectus excavatum deformity treated with Bio-Alcamid. Results highlight the successful treatment of gel migration with liposuction, which has not been recommended by the manufacturer nor reported in the literature to date.

▶ Bio-Alcamid is a permanent injectable soft tissue filler for the correction of contour and soft tissue deformities. It is composed of water (96%) with synthetic polymeric polyalkylimide (4%) and has been described as an injectable endoprosthesis. Reported complications include infection, migration, and capsule formation, which are treated by direct excision of the product. Although not currently available in the United States, it may be encountered in patients who travel out of the country for a procedure. Judging from this case report, liposuction may be a useful alternative for removal of Bio- Alcamid if the product has migrated.

K. A. Gutowski, MD

Treatment of Overweight Patients by Radiofrequency-Assisted Liposuction (RFAL) for Aesthetic Reshaping and Skin Tightening

Hurwitz D, Smith D (Univ of Pittsburgh Med School, PA)
Aesthetic Plast Surg 36:62-71, 2012

Background.—Patients with massive volume or skin laxity typically are not ideal candidates for liposuction treatment due to the excess amounts of loose skin after the procedure. The feasibility, safety, and efficacy of a novel radiofrequency device (BodyTite system) for radiofrequency-assisted liposuction (RFAL) were prospectively evaluated with overweight and weight loss patients.

Methods.—In this study, 17 women with an average aspirated volume of 1,759 ml in the arms, abdomen, or thighs were treated. The treatment technique is described with the resulting weight, circumferential, and contraction measurements collected at a follow-up assessment after 6 and 12 weeks. Three-dimensional scanning was used to document volume changes in selected cases. Patient satisfaction also was recorded. Body contour and area tightening results were evident for all the patients, with high posttreatment satisfaction. Skin contraction was significant at 6 weeks and continued past 12 weeks of follow-up evaluation.

Results.—On the average, after 12 weeks, patients had lost 6.2% of their original abdominal circumference, 4.4% of their original thigh circumference, and 9.2% of their original arm circumference. The mean vertical contraction was 7.9% for the abdomen, 3.6% for the thighs, and 2.4% for the arms. The maximum results showed a circumference loss of 16.5% for the abdomen, 11.4% for the thighs, and 17.7% for the arms. The maximum vertical contraction was 15.7% for the abdomen, 7.4% for the thighs, and 3.3% for the arms. The average follow-up period was 13.3 months (range, 3—26 months).

Conclusion.—The RFAL approach is a viable means of energy-assisted liposuction for overweight and massive weight loss patients. Significant volumes of fat can be removed safely and effectively with improved contour and clinically significant skin tightening.

▶ The patients included in this study had mild to moderate loose skin with fat excess and were overweight, had sustained massive weight loss (MWL), or had body-contouring surgery after MWL. It was expected that they would experience undesirable skin laxity after traditional liposuction. For this reason, radiofrequency-assisted liposuction (RFAL) was considered with the hope of improved posttreatment skin contraction. The RFAL device (BodyTite) is described in this article.

Although the objective results show improved measurements, suggesting skin contraction, the subjective assessment of before-treatment and after-treatment patient images is less convincing. Skin and soft tissue contour irregularities are present, and in some cases, the results look no different from what could be expected after traditional liposuction. As these patients were selected based on their high likelihood of having skin laxity after liposuction, perhaps offering RFAL (or other energy-assisted liposuction procedures) may be worthwhile, in the hope of some skin improvement.

K. A. Gutowski, MD

Correction of Liposuction Sequelae by Autologous Fat Transplantation
Pereira LH, Nicaretta B, Sterodimas A (LH Clinic, Rio de Janeiro, Brazil; Policlinca Geral, Rio de Janeiro, Brazil; Carlos Chagas Post-Graduate Med Inst, Rio de Janeiro, Brazil)
Aesthetic Plast Surg 35:1000-1008, 2011

Background.—In many countries, liposuction is the most frequently performed aesthetic procedure. Although lipo-suction has been considered a safe surgical procedure, reports indicate that it can have significant sequelae. Irregularities ranging from "oversuctioning" to bumpy skin and asymmetries result from inadequate experience of the surgeon.

Methods.—A total of 57 consecutive female patients were operated on from June 2005 to June 2007. The age distribution of the patients ranged from 22 to 53 years, with a mean of 34.2 years. All the patients that were included in the study had undergone from one to three liposuction procedures. Overall satisfaction with the body appearance after autologous fat transplantation for correction of post-liposuction irregularities was rated on a scale of 1−5, where 1 is poor, 2 is fair, 3 is good, 4 is very good, and 5 is excellent.

Results.—The total amount of clean adipose tissue transplanted varied from 14 to 120 ml. There were no cases of liponecrosis, which developed in the grafted area, and no liponecrotic lumps were palpated on postoperative evaluation on any operated cases. There were no cases of cellulitis at the donor or grafted area, no deep vein thrombosis, and no pulmonary embolism. There were nine cases that needed one additional session of fat grafting of 5−35 ml. Seven of those cases needed further fat grafting on the abdominal area and the remaining two needed further grafting of the infragluteal depressions. At 12 months, 68% reported that their appearance after autologous fat grafting was "very good" to "excellent" and 23% responded that their appearance was "good." Only 9% of patients thought their appearance was less than good.

Conclusion.—With the overall acceptance of aesthetic surgery increasing and the number of patients undergoing liposuction increasing, it is likely that plastic surgeons will see more patients requesting secondary contour surgery in the future. The key to successful autologous fat grafting is familiarity with the technique, recognizing its limitations, and understanding the goals of the patient. This study has shown that the patient satisfaction rate observed after autologous fat transplantation produces aesthetically acceptable results in correcting post liposuction deformities.

▶ Revision of liposuction contour deformities is typically done at least 6 months after the procedure to allow for scar softening and edema resolution. Waiting a full year, if possible, may allow for even better soft tissue quality and easier treatment. Fat grafts may be the best choice for improvement of depressed areas, and for smaller cases, this can be done as an office procedure using local anesthesia. The optimal fat graft harvesting, preparation, and injection methods have not been agreed on. In many cases, simple syringe aspiration and gravity sedimentation or mild centrifugation to remove the nonfat components is enough to obtain fat for correction of isolated defects. For larger defects, more than 1 treatment may be needed. Depending on the extent of the initial deformity, scarring, and skin quality, complete improvement may not be possible, so patient expectations should be realistic. Overall, the 12-month satisfaction rate in this study supports fat transplantation to correct postliposuction defects.

K. A. Gutowski, MD

Improving Outcomes in Upper Arm Liposuction: Adding Radiofrequency-Assisted Liposuction to Induce Skin Contraction

Duncan DI (Plastic Surgical Associates of Fort Collins, CO)
Aesthet Surg J 32:84-95, 2012

Background.—Brachioplasty is frequently recommended for patients with more skin laxity than subcutaneous fat. However, many patients are reluctant to accept a visible scar that will affect the activity of the upper arm or clothing choices. Traditional liposuction is effective when minimal skin laxity is present, but the dual problems of postoperative residual skin laxity and unsatisfactory contour irregularities are common when upper arm skin laxity is the chief complaint.

Objectives.—The author investigates the degree of skin contraction resulting from treatment with radiofrequency-assisted liposuction (RFAL) and attempts to determine whether, after long-term follow-up, the classification of upper arm deformities and their corresponding treatment protocols can be refined to offer patients with prominent skin laxity an alternative to traditional brachioplasty.

Methods.—A prospective, institutional review board—approved pilot study was planned with 12 consecutive patients who presented to the author's private clinic for treatment of upper arm laxity. Patients were included only if they were categorized as Stage 2b, 3, or 4 according to the El Khatib and Teimourian system. Based on the "pinch" test and the vertical measurement of skin distal to the bicipital groove as described by El Khatib, a novel caliper was devised to quantify the shortening of the pendulous volar skin. Treatment regions were tattooed prior to surgery and measurements from a Vectra system (Canfield Scientific, Inc., Fairfield, New Jersey) confirmed the preoperative surface area. All patients were treated with the BodyTite device (Invasix, Inc., Yokneam, Israel). No patient underwent skin resection in the volar treatment region. Skin contraction was measured at one year posttreatment. Statistical analysis was conducted with a paired *t*-test.

Results.—One year after treatment with RFAL, the mean surface area reduction in the volar upper arm region was 33.5% bilaterally. The mean degree of pendulous vertical "hang" shortening was 50% bilaterally. Statistical analysis showed a *P* value of >.001 for both measurements.

Conclusions.—Treatment with RFAL achieved statistically significant skin contraction in the upper arm region. Patients in categories 2b and 4 were successfully treated with RFAL instead of traditional brachioplasty (which is recommended by the current classification system). Category 3 patients, however, did require a short-scar brachioplasty procedure to obtain satisfactory results (Fig 11).

▶ Contouring options for the upper arm can be challenging in patients who already have skin laxity or are expected to have skin excess after liposuction. Unlike other body regions, skin excision in the arms tends to leave less favorable and more visible scars. The newer energy-based body contouring devices may

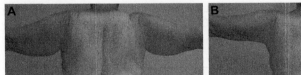

FIGURE 11.—(A) This 53-year-old woman presented with no weight loss, lipodystrophy, and skin excess. (B) One year after radiofrequency-assisted liposuction to both upper arms. (Reprinted from Duncan DI, Improving outcomes in upper arm liposuction: adding radiofrequency-assisted liposuction to induce skin contraction. *Aesthet Surg J.* 2012;32:84-95, with permission from The American Society for Aesthetic Plastic Surgery, Inc.)

offer an option for those patients who have mild to moderate laxity, are not accepting of a brachioplasty scar, but are willing to accept a more modest improvement in their result. These devices rely on laser, ultrasound, or radiofrequency energy to not only disrupt fat cells but also to increase connective tissue temperature and thereby cause collagen formation and tissue tightening.

Radiofrequency-assisted liposuction (RFAL) using the BodyTite is an invasive technique using an internal cannula with a tip that emits simultaneous radiofrequency (RF) energy and suction, as well as an overlying external electrode that reflects heat into the dermis of the skin in the treatment region. An "ironing" motion is used to heat the tissue in the region needing fat emulsification and skin contraction. The RF energy results in fat coagulation and liquefaction and also causes the fibrous septae surrounding the fat globules to contract.

The use of RF energy in liposuction does require additional time in each treatment area and more care to prevent complications in addition to having a steeper learning curve. There are also additional costs related to investing in the technology and in machine maintenance. The results do seem to offer a better outcome in selected patients compared with what would be expected with traditional liposuction (Fig 11) but a direct comparison of RFAL with other forms of liposuction was not done. Overall, this technology may be useful for borderline liposuction candidates. However, there are little data comparing the other invasive and noninvasive options for skin tightening. Cost, ease of use, and other practice-specific factors should be considered before considering this and other similar devices.

K. A. Gutowski, MD

6   Breast

General

Aesthetic Subunit of the Breast: An Analysis of Women's Preference and Clinical Implications

Bailey SH, Saint-Cyr M, Oni G, et al (Univ of Texas Southwestern Med Ctr, Dallas)
Ann Plast Surg 68:240-245, 2012

Patient satisfaction in breast surgery is dependent on achieving a balance among all aesthetic subunits. The purpose of this study is to identify which subunit of the breast women consider important and correlate this clinically to improve patient satisfaction following breast surgery.

A total of 313 subjects (ages, 20–80) were surveyed using a 25-point survey instrument collected via a telemedicine form. The data was analyzed to determine clinical significance.

Of the subjects, 63% selected the upper inner quadrant as the most important subunit. Furthermore, 66% of the subjects indicated defects located in this region would lead them to seek operative intervention and this was consistent for all subgroups. Based on these results, defects in the upper inner quadrant of the breast are more likely to cause patient dissatisfaction. Patient outcomes following surgery can be enhanced by restoring volume and minimizing scars in this upper medial subunit of the breast.

▶ Understanding a patient's perspective on breast appearance can help achieve higher patient satisfaction and decrease revisional procedures. In aesthetic breast surgery, explaining the dynamics and limitations of breast implants and breast cleavage to patients should be part of the educational process. In reconstructive breast surgery, a focus on replacing tissue in the inner upper quadrant is also critical to obtain a good result. Secondary fat grafting is becoming a common technique in correcting defects in this area.

K. A. Gutowski, MD

Duration of Antibiotics after Microsurgical Breast Reconstruction Does Not Change Surgical Infection Rate

Liu DZ, Dubbins JA, Louie O, et al (Univ of Washington School of Medicine, Seattle)
Plast Reconstr Surg 129:362-367, 2012

Background.—Infection rates for breast surgery are 3 to 15 percent, higher than average for a clean surgical procedure. Preoperative and postoperative antibiotics have lowered infection rates in other surgical groups, yet there is no consensus on postoperative prophylactic antibiotic use in microsurgical breast reconstruction.

Methods.—A retrospective review of consecutive patients who underwent autologous breast reconstruction between 2006 and 2009 was performed. Specific risk factors for autologous reconstruction were reviewed, including medical comorbidities, irradiation, and chemotherapy history. Data were collected on type and duration of prophylactic antibiotics. A prospective cohort of patients who received only 24 hours of postoperative antibiotics was identified. The incidence of surgical-site infections was measured using Centers for Disease Control and Prevention criteria.

Results.—A total of 256 patients with 360 microvascular breast reconstructions who received both preoperative and postoperative prophylactic antibiotics were analyzed. The overall surgical-site infection rate was 17.2 percent (44 of 256 patients). Surgical-site infection was correlated with increased age, tobacco use, and prior radiation. Duration of postoperative antibiotic use did not differ in those patients who developed surgical-site infections (6.2 versus 7.7 days; $p = 0.19$). Eighty-two patients (32 percent) received only 24 hours of postoperative antibiotics, while 174 (68 percent) received more than 24 hours of antibiotics for a median duration of 10 days. There was no difference in the overall surgical-site infection rate in those who received more than 24 hours of antibiotics (19.5 versus 15.5 percent; $p = 0.47$).

Conclusion.—There was no reduction in the overall surgical-site infection rate among autologous breast reconstruction patients who received postoperative antibiotic prophylaxis for more than 24 hours.

Clinical Question/Level of Evidence.—Therapeutic, III.

▶ One could ask several questions about this study and others like it. Why is the rate of breast cancer surgery as high and as varied as 3% to 15% and are those rates really inevitable? The Cochrane study by Cunningham et al[1] found that preoperative antibiotics in breast cancer patients significantly reduced the risk of postoperative wound infection, but that perioperative antibiotics did not alter the risk over the use of no antibiotics. These authors state that they gave preoperative antibiotics within 60 minutes of the skin incision, but does that mean they were preoperative or could the skin incision have been made prior to the dosing? What is the rate of wound infection in delayed breast reconstruction, with breast implants, in patients who have not undergone chemotherapy or radiotherapy, and should it be 10-fold greater than in patients undergoing routine breast augmentation? Is there a difference in surgical site infection between patients undergoing delayed breast reconstruction with implants versus autologous tissue? The major problem with this study is there was no agreed upon protocol that set the time for the administration of the antibiotics, the particular antibiotic used, standardization regarding the tissues used for reconstruction, and the length of time for the use of postoperative antibiotics. Finally, the numbers are just too small when broken down into subcategories to be sure whether there was or was not an effect of using preoperative and postoperative antibiotics versus just preoperative antibiotics. It seems to me that these questions could be addressed by developing a standardized multi-institutional, prospective randomized, controlled study with adequate power for conclusions to be generally accepted as significant.

S. H. Miller, MD

Reference

1. Cunningham M, Bunn F, Handscomb K. Prophylactic antibiotics to prevent surgical site infection after breast cancer surgery. *Cochrane Database Syst Rev.* 2006;(2):CCD005360.

Duration of Antibiotics after Microsurgical Breast Reconstruction Does Not Change Surgical Infection Rate
Liu DZ, Dubbins JA, Louie O, et al (Univ of Washington School of Medicine, Seattle)
Plast Reconstr Surg 129:362-367, 2012

Background.—Infection rates for breast surgery are 3 to 15 percent, higher than average for a clean surgical procedure. Preoperative and postoperative antibiotics have lowered infection rates in other surgical groups, yet there is no consensus on postoperative prophylactic antibiotic use in microsurgical breast reconstruction.

Methods.—A retrospective review of consecutive patients who underwent autologous breast reconstruction between 2006 and 2009 was performed. Specific risk factors for autologous reconstruction were reviewed, including medical comorbidities, irradiation, and chemotherapy history. Data were collected on type and duration of prophylactic antibiotics. A prospective cohort of patients who received only 24 hours of postoperative antibiotics was identified. The incidence of surgical-site infections was measured using Centers for Disease Control and Prevention criteria.

Results.—A total of 256 patients with 360 microvascular breast reconstructions who received both preoperative and postoperative prophylactic antibiotics were analyzed. The overall surgical-site infection rate was 17.2 percent (44 of 256 patients). Surgical-site infection was correlated with increased age, tobacco use, and prior radiation. Duration of postoperative antibiotic use did not differ in those patients who developed surgical-site infections (6.2 versus 7.7 days; $p = 0.19$). Eighty-two patients (32 percent) received only 24 hours of postoperative antibiotics, while 174 (68 percent) received more than 24 hours of antibiotics for a median duration of 10 days. There was no difference in the overall surgical-site infection rate in those who received more than 24 hours of antibiotics (19.5 versus 15.5 percent; $p = 0.47$).

Conclusion.—There was no reduction in the overall surgical-site infection rate among autologous breast reconstruction patients who received postoperative antibiotic prophylaxis for more than 24 hours.

Clinical Question/Level of Evidence.—Therapeutic, III.

▶ The authors report there was no difference in the surgical site infection rate for patients who receive postoperative antibiotic prophylaxis for greater than 24 hours following autologous breast reconstruction compared with those who received only 24 hours of postoperative antibiotic prophylaxis. This is a nicely done retrospective study. The subgroups are well analyzed and the downside of continued antibiotic use outlined. The need for a prospective study is evident so we can begin to use evidence basis, not personal bias.

D. J. Smith, Jr, MD

Mastopexy and Reduction

Increasing Age Impairs Outcomes in Breast Reduction Surgery
Shermak MA, Chang D, Buretta K, et al (The Johns Hopkins Med Institutions, Baltimore, MD)
Plast Reconstr Surg 128:1182-1187, 2011

Background.—Although multiple breast reduction outcomes studies have been performed, none has specifically identified the impact of advanced age. The authors aimed to study the impact of age on breast reduction outcome.

Methods.—Medical records for all patients billed for Current Procedural Terminology code 19318 over the past 10 years (1999 to 2009) at a large academic institution were analyzed under an institutional review board—approved protocol. A total of 1192 consecutive patients underwent 2156 reduction mammaplasties performed by 17 plastic surgeons over a 10-year period. Breast reduction techniques included inferior pedicle/Wise pattern in 1250 patients (58.9 percent), medial pedicle/Wise pattern in 360 (16.9 percent), superior pedicle/nipple graft in 305 (14.4 percent), superior pedicle/vertical pattern in 206 (9.7 percent), and liposuction in three (0.14 percent). The average patient age was 36 years. Age groups were divided into younger than 40 years, 40 to 50 years, and older than 50 years. Multiple logistic regression analysis was performed to identify significant relationships.

Results.—Women older than 50 years more likely experienced infection (odds ratio, 2.7; $p = 0.003$), with trends toward wound healing problems (odds ratio, 1.6; $p = 0.09$) and reoperative wound débridement (odds ratio, 5.1; $p = 0.07$). There was a trend toward infection in women aged 40 to 50 years (odds ratio, 1.7; $p = 0.08$). Advanced age did not exacerbate fat necrosis or seroma development.

Conclusions.—Age older than 50 years impairs breast reduction outcomes, particularly infection, and may negatively impact wound healing. Hormonal deficiency may partially account for this finding.
Clinical Question/Level of Evidence.—Risk, IV.

▶ This carefully done study provides the plastic surgeon with information that should help in counseling older patients about breast reduction surgery and may also heighten the surgeon's awareness of possible complications in this age group. However, the information is not likely to change decisions regarding the appropriateness of breast reduction in patients over age 50. The evidence (in many prior studies) of documented benefits of the procedure in all age groups appears to clearly outweigh the concerns about infection (statistically significant in this study), wound healing (a trend without statistical significance), or reoperation (again, a trend). Reduction even after age 60 (not studied separately in this article) can still be justified in patients with good health and appropriate symptoms of macromastia. The surgeon should use the information in this study to warn patients of possible increased complication rates in those aged 50 and older and give patients the option to decline the surgery if their concerns are great. The suggestion that exogenous hormone use combats infection is interesting and warrants further investigation.

R. L. Ruberg, MD

A Retrospective Photometric Study of 82 Published Reports of Mastopexy and Breast Reduction
Swanson E (Private Practice, Leawood, KS)
Plast Reconstr Surg 128:1282-1301, 2011

Background.—Numerous publications claim to improve breast projection and upper pole fullness after mastopexy or breast reduction. Fascial sutures and "autoaugmentation" with local flaps are advocated. However, there is no objective evidence that these efforts are effective. The author has proposed a measuring system to quantitate results. Not only is this system useful for assessing one's own results, but it may also be used to assess and compare results in published studies.

Methods.—Eighty-two international publications on mastopexies and breast reductions were analyzed. The studies were grouped by technique: inverted-T (superior/medial, central, and inferior pedicles), vertical, periareolar, inframammary, lateral, and "other." Measurements were made using the definitions and terminology reported separately and included breast projection, upper pole projection, lower pole level, nipple level, breast convexity, breast parenchymal ratio, and lower pole ratio. Areola shape was assessed.

Results.—Breast projection and upper pole projection were not increased significantly by any of the mastopexy/reduction procedures or by the use of fascial sutures or autoaugmentation techniques. Nipple overelevation was common (41.9 percent). The incidence of the teardrop areola deformity (53.8 percent) was significantly higher ($p < 0.001$) in patients treated with the open technique of nipple placement. There was no significant difference in results when compared by follow-up times, resection weights, year of publication, or geographic region.

Conclusions.—Existing mastopexy/reduction techniques do not significantly increase breast projection or upper pole projection. Fascial sutures and autoaugmentation techniques are ineffective. Nipple overelevation and the teardrop areola deformity are common problems and should be avoided.

▶ There is nothing like a thoughtful study with carefully performed measurements to refute long-standing but unsubstantiated opinions and impressions. For many years, a great variety of techniques has been promoted for improving breast projection and upper-pole fullness after mastectomy, including sutures, flaps, muscle slings, tissue rearrangements, and so on. In virtually every instance, the results were "documented" by visual impression rather than precise measurement. Provided that the reader is willing to accept the author's personal measurements and his quantitative techniques as valid determinants of projection and fullness, the article effectively discredits the conclusions of all previous studies claiming improvement after mastopexy. However, this consideration does not invalidate previous methods; it only denies the claims of improvement. So if a mastopexy procedure effectively "lifts" the breast and maintains existing projection and upper-pole fullness, the surgeon may still consider the procedure to be effective, and one that accomplishes the usual patient's major objectives—to reduce or eliminate breast sagging. The author cautions about overelevation cannot be overemphasized: once a nipple/areola complex is too high, there is virtually no good way to restore normal relationships without incurring significant scarring or risking continued deformity.

R. L. Ruberg, MD

Does Knowledge of the Initial Technique Affect Outcomes after Repeated Breast Reduction?

Ahmad J, McIsaac SM, Lista F (Univ of Ottawa, Ontario, Canada)
Plast Reconstr Surg 129:11-18, 2012

Background.—This article examines outcomes following repeated breast reduction using vertical scar reduction mammaplasty. The results of performing repeated breast reduction in patients for whom operative records were available for the previous breast reduction were compared with those for whom these records could not be obtained.

Methods.—A retrospective review of all patients who underwent repeated breast reduction for recurrent symptomatic mammary hypertrophy, inadequate volume reduction during the primary operation, and significant postoperative breast volume asymmetry was performed.

Results.—Twenty-five patients had repeated breast reduction. The initial technique was known in 13 patients and unknown in 12 patients. The average total reduction per breast (including liposuction) was 658 g (range, 30 to 1150 g). Liposuction was used more often in cases for which the initial technique was unknown ($p = 0.000$). No patients experienced necrosis of the nipple-areola complex, and there was no significant difference in the complication rates between patients for whom the previous pedicle was known versus those in whom it was unknown ($p = 0.220$).

Conclusions.—Using vertical scar reduction mammaplasty, repeated breast reduction is a safe procedure, even when the initial technique is unknown. A vertically oriented, inferior wedge excision of tissue can be safely excised, irrespective of the initial pedicle. For patients with ptosis in whom the nipple-areola complex needs to be transposed superiorly, a carefully planned and de-epithelialized superior pedicle should be used. In addition, liposuction is an important adjunct to achieve volume reduction, while limiting the amount of dissection during repeated breast reduction.

Clinical Question/Level of Evidence.—Therapeutic, IV.

▶ This article provides useful information about appropriate techniques for repeat reduction mammaplasty. Conventional wisdom has been that the surgeon should determine (from the prior operative note) which technique was used previously, and then use the same technique to minimize the chances of complications. These authors defy conventional wisdom and apply the same technique—vertical scar breast reduction—to all cases, with excellent results. Often the greatest concern in repeat breast reduction is nipple-areola complex vascular compromise, leading to necrosis. This problem was not encountered in this series, perhaps because the nipple often remains at an elevated position, even if breast hypertrophy has recurred or "fall-out" of the inferior portion of the breast has occurred. As a result of this higher nipple position, the short superior pedicle, as would be required in the vertical scar reduction technique, should maximize viability of the nipple. The addition of liposuction, as opposed to more aggressive tissue excision, probably increases the chances of avoiding complications. Therefore, in the hands of these authors the vertical scar technique was almost uniformly successful irrespective of the previously used technique.

R. L. Ruberg, MD

Augmentation and Silicone

Breast Augmentation Using Preexpansion and Autologous Fat Transplantation: A Clinical Radiographic Study

Del Vecchio DA, Bucky LP (Back Bay Plastic Surgery, Boston, MA)
Plast Reconstr Surg 127:2441-2450, 2011

Background.—Despite the increased popularity of fat grafting of the breasts, there remain unanswered questions. There is currently no standard for technique or data regarding long-term volume maintenance with this procedure. Because of the sensitive nature of breast tissue, there is a need for radiographic evaluation, focusing on volume maintenance and on tissue viability. This study was designed to quantify the long-term volume maintenance of mature adipocyte fat grafting for breast augmentation using recipient-site preexpansion.

Methods.—This is a prospective examination of 25 patients in 46 breasts treated with fat grafting for breast augmentation from 2007 to 2009. Indications included micromastia, postexplantation deformity, tuberous breast deformity, and Poland syndrome. Preexpansion using the BRAVA device was used in all patients. Fat was processed using low−g-force centrifugation. Patients had preoperative and 6-month postoperative three-dimensional volumetric imaging and/or magnetic resonance imaging to quantify breast volume.

Results.—All women had a significant increase in breast volume (range, 60 to 200 percent) at 6 months, as determined by magnetic resonance imaging ($n = 12$), and all had breasts that were soft and natural in appearance and feel. Magnetic resonance imaging examinations postoperatively revealed no new oil cysts or breast masses.

Conclusions.—Preexpansion of the breast allows for megavolume (>300 cc) grafting with reproducible, long-lasting results that can be achieved in less than 2 hours. These data can serve as a benchmark with which to evaluate the safety and efficacy of other core technology strategies in fat grafting. The authors believe preexpansion is useful for successful megavolume fat grafting to the breast.

▶ This article provides valuable evidence regarding the effectiveness of breast augmentation accomplished purely with fat transplantation but still leaves many unanswered questions about the specific steps used by the authors to achieve their results. The long-term (6-month) postoperative imaging studies confirm the persistence of transplanted fat in the operated breasts. The photographs show impressive, natural results. The authors carefully detail their treatment approach: presurgical pre-expansion, simple fat preparation, and large volume injections. The study shows that large-volume injection is effective and well tolerated. However, there is less scientific evidence for the need for pre-expansion or for the specific fat preparation methods used by the authors. One can conclude that what they do works. But is it necessary? Maybe. The authors provide ample theoretical evidence supporting the need for the various steps in their approach. But they correctly note that more scientific study is needed before concluding that the steps that they take yield results better than those accomplished without pre-expansion or with different fat preparation techniques. Bottom line: what they do does work, and works well.

R. L. Ruberg, MD

The Influence of Career Stage, Practice Type and Location, and Physician's Sex on Surgical Practices Among Board-Certified Plastic Surgeons Performing Breast Augmentation

Naidu NS, Patrick PA (Plastic Surgeon in Private Practice in New York; Winthrop Univ Hosp, Mineola, NY)
Aesthet Surg J 31:941-952, 2011

Background.—Breast augmentation is the most commonly performed cosmetic surgical procedure in the United States, but surgeon preferences in terms of technique and postoperative care regimen vary widely.

Objectives.—The authors investigated the influence of career stage, practice type and location, and physician's sex on surgical technique preferences among board-certified plastic surgeons performing breast augmentation.

Methods.—In October 2009, an online survey was e-mailed to all active members of the American Society of Plastic Surgeons practicing within the United States. Response frequencies were calculated and correlated with surgeon demographics.

Results.—From the pool of 4737 respondents, 898 responses were received (18.9%). Surgeons performing breast augmentation were more frequently male, between 46 and 65 years old, and had practiced for at least 20 years in solo private practice in a suburban setting. Surgical volume most frequently consisted of 10% to 25% cosmetic surgery, with 10 to 50 breast augmentations performed per year. Surgeons in practice for five years or less were more likely to use smooth, round silicone gel-filled implants, to select implants smaller than 300 cc, to use the dual-plane pocket, and to recommend yearly follow-up. Surgeons in practice for more than 20 years were more likely to select saline implants, utilize the subglandular plane, perform closed capsulotomy, and place drains. Surgeons at academic centers performed fewer breast augmentation surgeries and placed smaller implants than those in private practice, while surgeons in suburban locations performed more breast augmentations than those in urban or rural locations. Surgeons in the West performed the greatest number of augmentations, although the largest-sized implants were placed in the Southwest. Compared with men, women surgeons appeared significantly less likely to use saline implants, were less likely to perform more than 100 breast augmentations per year, and were significantly more likely to place implants less than 300 cc.

Conclusions.—Surgical preferences were associated with years in practice and included differences in technique and postoperative care. Practice location was associated with differences in procedural volume, implant size, incision location, and recommended follow-up time, while practice type was related to surgical volume, implant size, implant location, and percentage of cosmetic surgery performed.

▶ In an era of evidence-based medicine (EBM), it would be expected that all surgeons would have similar rates of specific practice patterns if presented with similar patients. Yet this survey shows striking differences in breast augmentation preferences when by a surgeon's years in practice, gender, and practice setting are compared. This suggests that influences other than EBM affect a surgeon's approach.

Surprisingly, less than 10% of surgeons used an objective method (Tebbett's TEPID system) of implant size selection. Likewise, surgeons who relied on the patient's choice as the determining factor in selecting implant size were significantly more likely to place implants larger than 350 cc, compared with those who relied on their own judgment for selection. Almost one-third prescribed Accolate, Singulair, or other medications for treatment of capsular contracture despite limited studies of effectiveness. One in 5 surgeons used Betadine solution pocket irrigation even though the Food and Drug Administration and implant package inserts advise against it. Not surprisingly, surgeons in practice for 5 years or less showed a tendency to be both conservative and cautious, as demonstrated by their tendency to place smaller implants, change the implant pocket for the first instance of capsular contracture, and recommend yearly follow-up.

As the authors point out, these finds suggest that surgeons are more likely to retain the techniques learned during their training or early in their careers, suggesting that they rely more on their personal experience than the current literature as their careers advance. For this reason, each of us should actively seek out current and relevant educational opportunities for improving our practice patterns, rather than rely solely on personal experience and, at times, outdated training.

K. A. Gutowski, MD

The "Triple-Plane Technique" for Breast Augmentation

Bracaglia R, Gentileschi S, Fortunato R (Università Cattolica Sacro Cuore, Rome, Italy; Casa di Cura Villa Stuart, Rome, Italy)
Aesthetic Plast Surg 35:859-865, 2011

Breast augmentation is one of the most frequently performed aesthetic surgery procedures. In the United States, it is the second most commonly performed aesthetic surgery procedure among women, according to the American Society of Aesthetic Plastic Surgery statistics. Different choices available to the surgeon deal with the pocket plane, the skin incisions, and the type of implant. This report describes the results from a retrospective review of the authors' experience with the "triple-plane technique" and its different indications according to breast types. Findings have shown that this technique is suitable for many different types, shapes, and sizes of breasts; that it offers very good and natural results; and particularly, that these results last over time.

▶ The authors present a new approach to submuscular breast augmentation. The most common technique for this type of augmentation involves inferior release of the pectoralis major muscle, allowing the muscle to rise superiorly. Then, when the implant is placed in its pocket, the upper portion of the implant lies posterior to the muscle, and the lower portion lies posterior to the gland, thus, creating a dual plane pocket. The senior author of this article starts essentially with a total submuscular pocket, then splits the muscle transversely at the level of the nipple and allows the muscle to gape open. When the implant is placed, it is submuscular in the upper portion, subglandular in the middle portion, and again submuscular at the lower pole. They call this a *triple plane* approach, although only 2 different planes are used. The *triple* refers to the fact that there are 3 separate zones of implant position. The main advantage claimed for this approach is better support of the lower pole of the implant with less chance for inferior migration or implant palpability compared with the dual plane approach, which leaves only skin and gland supporting the prosthesis at the bottom of the breast. Another suggested advantage is less flattening of the central portion of the implant by overlying pectoralis muscle. The results shown in the article seem quite good. Time and more studies by other investigators are needed to confirm the suggested superiority of this technique over the standard dual plane approach.

R. L. Ruberg, MD

Subpectoral and Precapsular Implant Repositioning Technique: Correction of Capsular Contracture and Implant Malposition

Lee HK, Jin US, Lee YH (Image Plastic Surgery Clinic, Seoul, Republic of Korea; Seoul Natl Univ Hosp, Seoul, Republic of Korea)
Aesth Plast Surg 35:1126-1132, 2011

Background.—Although capsule formation is a natural-healing process following breast augmentation using implants, a contracted capsule around a poorly positioned implant can act as an obstacle during the corrective procedure to reposition the implant. The ideal treatment of capsular contracture is removal of the capsule and covering the implant with a healthy envelope without scar tissue. However, total capsulectomy in the submuscular space may be difficult, especially if the capsule is firmly attached to the chest wall. This situation may require a highly skilled technique because aggressive capsulectomy could injure the intercostal muscles and vasculature and cause further complications such as pneumothorax. Therefore, the authors have developed a new, less traumatic method of leaving the capsule behind the new implant.

Method.—From February 2001 through February 2009, the authors treated 74 patients (139 breasts) using a subpectoral, precapsular implant repositioning technique. These patients suffered from capsular contracture or implant malposition after submuscular breast augmentation. The technique is composed of three parts. First, a plane was developed between the anterior wall of the capsule and the posterior surface of the pectoralis major muscle using a periareolar or inframammary approach. After removing the previous implant, the anterior wall of the capsule was fully released from the posterior surface of the pectoralis major muscle and fixed to the posterior wall of the capsule which adhered to the chest wall. The new implant was inserted into the developed subpectoral space, anterior to the capsule.

Results.—The mean age of the patients was 31 years (range = 24–52) and the time between the primary and the secondary augmentation was

42 months (range = 4 months to 12 years). The range for follow-up was from 12 months to 5 years. Median follow-up was 26 months. Postoperative complications included two cases of hematoma but no cases of infection, muscle distortion, or double-bubble deformity.

Conclusion.—This technique is a valid alternative treatment for capsular contracture or malpositioned implant after breast augmentation surgery. It may be less traumatic than the conventional method of total capsulectomy. In addition, this technique reduces the relapse rate of capsular contracture significantly compared to a partial capsulectomy or capsulotomy as the new implant is inserted into a scar tissue-free environment. Good aesthetic results and patient satisfaction was achieved using this method. In our experience, this novel technique is a good alternative method of correcting complications of submuscular implant augmentation.

▶ The authors propose a new approach to repositioning breast implants in patients with capsular contracture after submuscular augmentation. Their premise is that leaving the capsule in place reduces the chances of chest wall complications (eg, pneumothorax) versus when total capsulectomy is carried out before replacing the implant. Realistically, the chances of significant chest wall problems in patients undergoing capsulectomy after simple submuscular augmentation are low. Nevertheless, this approach may have some merit in simplifying the procedure and may perhaps be especially helpful in very thin patients. This approach may have a more important application in patients who require capsulectomy after postmastectomy reconstruction. In this circumstance, removal of the posterior wall of the capsule may indeed be more of a challenge, so an operation that simply leaves the entire capsule in place may reduce risks. The authors acknowledge that problems could occur because of leaving the capsule in place, and they address this possibility by closing the capsule with multiple sutures and leaving an opening inferiorly, which presumably reduces the chances of seroma or other permanent fluid collection. There is insufficient evidence to evaluate the long-term effectiveness of this particular treatment of potential seroma.

R. L. Ruberg, MD

Sensitivity of the Nipple-Areola Complex and Areolar Pain following Aesthetic Breast Augmentation in a Retrospective Series of 1200 Patients: Periareolar versus Submammary Incision
Araco A, Araco F, Sorge R, et al (Univ of Tor Vergata, Rome, Italy; Leicester Royal Infirmary, UK)
Plast Reconstr Surg 128:984-989, 2011

Background.—Different studies have investigated the anatomical and operative factors associated with alterations of nipple-areola complex sensitivity after aesthetic breast augmentation. The authors conducted a retrospective evaluation of a large series of patients to assess the risk factors that could be associated with such alterations.

Methods.—Data were collected retrospectively from the personal archive of the first author from May of 2004 to September of 2010. Excluded were those that underwent operations on the breast different from augmentation (i.e., breast reductions), augmentations associated with other operations that could influence the nipple-areola complex (e.g., mastopexy, lifting of the nipple, inverted nipple, reduction of the nipple, capsulectomy), breast revisions, breast implant replacements, or monolateral or nonsymmetrical augmentations.

Results.—The number of patients included in the study was 1222. The only factor associated with nipple-areola complex sensitivity alterations and areolar pain at 6 months was the type of skin incision used. Alterations were more present postoperatively with the periareolar than with the submammary incision (chi-square test, $p = 0.001$). The periareolar incision increased the risk of nipple-areola complex sensitivity alterations almost threefold and the risk of areolar pain by more than threefold.

Conclusions.—The type of skin incision adopted for breast augmentation seems to influence the occurrence of postoperative nipple-areola complex alterations of sensitivity or areolar pain. Although this affects a small percentage of patients, it is worth mentioning so that a more lucid informed consent and agreement to the operation can be achieved.

Clinical Question/Level of Evidence.—Therapeutic, III.

▶ Although there have been previous studies that evaluated the influence incision location has on postoperative nipple-areola sensation and pain after breast augmentation, this study provides information that may be more reliable than the earlier reviews because of the large number of patients (1222) studied. The clear message in this study is that an incision at the areolar border, for reasons that may seem obvious but are not documented, has the potential to reduce nipple sensation and increase nipple pain 6 months after surgery. It is important, however, to note that the actual number of patients who experienced these problems was quite low: there were only 55 patients (about 4.5%) who had reduced or absent sensation, and 68 patients (about 5.5%) who complained of at least some degree of pain. Strengths of this study include use of a standardized technique, all procedures were done by a single surgeon, and the results were controlled for implant location, implant size, and patient age, all of which did not have a measurable influence. Weaknesses include the study was retrospective, and the decreased sensation was determined by self-reporting, not objective measurement. The value of the study is the importance of providing another important detail to the patient in the preoperative period. It is not clear whether patients, given these data, including the actual incidence of problems, would prefer an incision that is potentially less visible (ie, the periareolar incision) or one that has a lower likelihood of sensation reduction and persistent nipple pain (the inframammary incision).

R. L. Ruberg, MD

Cancer and Reconstruction

Commonwealth of Massachusetts Board of Registration in Medicine Expert Panel on Immediate Implant-Based Breast Reconstruction Following Mastectomy for Cancer: Executive Summary, June 2011
Lee BT, the Massachusetts Board of Registration in Medicine Expert Panel on Immediate Implant-Based Breast Reconstruction following Mastectomy for Cancer (Beth Israel Deaconess Med Ctr, Boston, MA; et al)
J Am Coll Surg 213:800-805, 2011

Background.—An estimated 207,000 women in the United States received a new breast cancer diagnosis in 2010. Many require mastectomy and even more choose mastectomy to reduce their risk of local recurrence. Many women who have mastectomy will choose to have immediate implant-based reconstruction. With the Food and Drug Administration (FDA) reapproval of silicone implants and the introduction of various implant types and acellular dermal matric material, esthetic results are vastly improved. In early 2010 Massachusetts convened a statewide multidisciplinary expert panel to study the dynamic changes in this field, identify the best practices for implant-based reconstruction, and recommend a course of action for future practice and data collection efforts. Their report was summarized.

Patient Education and Informed Consent.—The panel recommends that providers develop a compassionate, patient-centered process for presenting treatment options and making decisions considering patient preferences. The weeks immediately after the woman is diagnosed are the most psychologically difficult for the patient. The provider must allow a period for building trust and understanding the patient's emotional status, values, knowledge, and desire to participate in the decision-making process. Providers must also consider patient values and preferences when discussing risks and benefits of the options, including the choice for no reconstruction. The panel also stresses that appropriate management of the patient's expectations for the reconstruction are important to the decision-making and informed consent process. Patients who take an active role in making decisions tend to be more satisfied with the result and have more positive outcomes. In shared decision-making, providers and patients share treatment decisions informed by the best evidence available and weighted according to the specifics of the individual patient. This is essential in the informed consent process for mastectomy and breast reconstruction. The shared decision-making process and the informed consent actions should be supported by multiple well-written, clinically accurate decision aids to give patients specific ideas about questions to ask and to allow them to learn at their own pace and at home. Informed consent is a process derived from the ethical and legal obligations of the provider toward the patient and includes the time needed for patients to accept the diagnosis. Aspects of informed consent include the nature of the decision or procedure; reasonable alternatives; relevant risks, benefits, and uncertainties for each alternative;

an assessment of whether the patient understands; and acceptance of the intervention by the patient.

Risk Factors, Technical Issues, and Perioperative Care.—The need for adjuvant radiotherapy is the primary consideration when deciding if the patient is a candidate for immediate breast reconstruction. If radiotherapy will be used, breast reconstruction should be delayed. Complications of breast reconstruction are more likely in the presence of smoking; obesity; radiation before, during, or after reconstruction; ischemic or necrotic mastectomy flaps after breast reconstruction; and neoadjuvant chemotherapy. Inherent risks also attend the use of implants, expanders, and acellular dermal matrix. Patients must be informed of these risks and the discussion documented. Infection prevention recommendations are consistent with those of the Massachusetts Healthcare Associated Infection Expert Panel. If the patient develops infection, aggressive, early surgical intervention and more liberal use of explantation are appropriate should antibiotic treatment not provoke an early response. Hospitals should develop a Focused Professional Practice Evaluation for surgeons to ensure competence and document appropriate training to perform breast reconstruction procedures. Included in this evaluation is having a surgeon experienced in breast reconstruction observe the applying surgeon and help track outcomes.

Improving Care.—Clinical data are collected to document breast reconstruction outcomes and assess treatment efficacy. In addition, a data collection system that meets best practice standards should be developed.

Conclusions.—The work of the Massachusetts panel continues. An advisory committee is tasked with developing a uniform data collection system. The panel's findings are also designed to be used to develop educational materials for patients.

▶ This is an excellent summary report from an expert multispecialty panel of physicians on the current status of immediate implant-based breast reconstruction following mastectomy in the state of Massachusetts. The group was led by a general surgeon and a plastic surgeon. Many of their recommendations have been expressed in individual reports, but the goals of the panel were to improve patient care through and evidence-based review of the literature and to identify best practices. I believe they have begun to accomplish their goals and would heartily recommend that they follow through on their plans to participate in the American College of Surgeons National Surgical Quality Improvement Program. The summary is worthwhile for all reconstructive breast surgeons to read and follow closely as new material is published by this group. I was particularly taken by and heartily agree with their suggestion that hospitals, in accord with suggestions made by The Joint Commission, should develop focused professional practice groups to evaluate the training and education as well as ongoing competence of those practicing breast reconstruction through the use of experienced observers and outcome data collection.

S. H. Miller, MD

Should we continue to consider obesity a relative contraindication for autologous microsurgical breast reconstruction?

Momeni A, Ahdoot MA, Kim RY, et al (Stanford Univ Med Ctr, Palo Alto, CA; Stanford Univ Med Ctr, CA)
J Plast Reconstr Aesthet Surg 65:420-425, 2012

Background.—Obesity is not only a causative factor for premature mortality, it has also been demonstrated to be associated with an increased postoperative complication rate. As such, it has traditionally been considered a relative contraindication to autologous breast reconstruction. The purpose of this study was to assess whether this recommendation is justified.

Methods.—A retrospective study was conducted analyzing the effect of obesity on complication rate after microsurgical autologous breast reconstruction using abdominal tissue. Patients undergoing breast reconstruction between November 2006 and February 2011 were included. In contrast to prior studies, only patients meeting criteria to undergo bariatric surgery were included in the study, thus, representing a particularly high-risk subset of patients (Group 1: BMI greater 40 kg/m^2; Group 2: BMI greater 35 kg/m^2 with co-morbidities).

Results.—A total of 42 breast reconstructions were performed in 28 patients who met inclusion criteria. Surgical complications were seen in a total of 9 patients ($p = 1.00$). All complications were successfully managed conservatively and did not prolong hospitalization. No differences were seen among study groups with respect to donor-site ($p = 0.57$) and recipient-site complications ($p = 1.00$). Of note, no partial or total flap loss was seen in this study.

Conclusions.—Obesity is associated with a relatively high risk of minor complications postoperatively. However, complications can typically be managed non-operatively and on an outpatient basis with fairly minimal patient morbidity. We believe that obesity should not be considered a relative contraindication to autologous microsurgical breast reconstruction. Patients should, however, be informed preoperatively about their higher risk of postoperative complications.

▶ The authors believe the traditional dogma that obesity represents a relative contraindication to autologous breast reconstruction does not hold true in light of recent studies. They do acknowledge that limitations to their study include the retrospective study design as well as limited number of patients. This is troubling. How can they make such a strong recommendation with such major shortcomings? At best, these results call for a prospective, randomized trial. Basing dogmatic recommendations on trials such as this may get us in trouble with future care.

D. J. Smith, Jr, MD

Breast Reconstruction with Free Tissue Transfer from the Abdomen in the Morbidly Obese

Jandali S, Nelson JA, Sonnad SS, et al (Univ of Pennsylvania Health System, Philadelphia)

Plast Reconstr Surg 127:2206-2213, 2011

Background.—There are national trends of increasing incidence of morbid obesity and autologous breast reconstruction with free tissue transfer from the abdomen. The purpose of this study was to assess the safety and efficacy of free flap breast reconstruction in the morbidly obese population.

Methods.—A retrospective review was conducted on all patients who underwent transverse rectus abdominis myocutaneous, deep inferior epigastric perforator, or superficial inferior epigastric artery flap breast reconstructions between July of 2006 and October of 2008. Data from all patients with a body mass index greater than 40 were compared with those of patients with a body mass index less than 40. A p value less than 0.05 was considered significant. Significant findings were then analyzed in a post hoc fashion to examine trends with increasing body mass index.

Results.—Four hundred four patients underwent 612 free flap breast reconstructions during the study period. Twenty-five of these patients (6 percent) had a body mass index greater than 40. The morbidly obese group had significantly higher rate of total flap loss ($p = 0.02$), total major postoperative complications ($p = 0.05$), and delayed wound healing ($p = 0.006$).

Conclusions.—Free flap breast reconstruction in the morbidly obese is associated with a higher risk of total flap loss, total major postoperative complications, and delayed abdominal wound healing. However, the overall incidence of complications is low, making free tissue transfer from the abdomen an acceptable method of breast reconstruction in this patient population.

▶ The real question about breast reconstruction in the morbidly obese patient is whether ANY form of reconstruction should be attempted. Unfortunately, these patients are poor candidates for simpler forms of reconstruction utilizing implants or tissue expanders because of size concerns—it simply is impossible in the truly morbidly obese patient to place an implant that creates anything other than a (relatively) very small breast. Furthermore, use of external prostheses is similarly problematic in these patients because the device is usually much too heavy for comfort. So the only real choices are no reconstruction or autogenous reconstruction (best done as a free flap). These authors make the case that free tissue transfer, even with its documented attendant complications of total flap loss and significant problems with abdominal wound healing, is worth the effort. It is important to remember in analyzing the results reported in this study that the authors are very technically adept surgeons with a very large case experience. Therefore, the individual surgeon must carefully weigh the options, thoroughly explain the potential risks, and arrive at a treatment plan after full patient participation in the decision process.

R. L. Ruberg, MD

Disparities in Reconstruction Rates After Mastectomy: Patterns of Care and Factors Associated With the Use of Breast Reconstruction in Southern California

Kruper L, Holt A, Xu XX, et al (City of Hope Natl Med Ctr, Duarte, CA)
Ann Surg Oncol 18:2158-2165, 2011

Background.—Many factors influence whether breast cancer patients undergo reconstruction after mastectomy. We sought to determine the patterns of care and variables associated with the use of breast reconstruction in Southern California.

Materials and Methods.—Postmastectomy reconstruction rates were determined from the California Office of Statewide Health Planning and Development (OSHPD) inpatient database from 2003 to 2007. International Classification of Disease-9 codes were used to identify patients undergoing reconstruction after mastectomy. Changes in reconstruction rates were examined by calendar year, age, race, type of insurance, and type of hospital using a chi-square test. Univariate and multivariate odds ratios (OR) with 95% confidence intervals (95% CI) were estimated for relative odds of immediate reconstruction versus mastectomy only.

Results.—In multivariate analysis, calendar year, age, race, type of insurance, and type of hospital were statistically significantly associated with use of reconstruction. The proportion of patients undergoing reconstruction rose from 24.8% in 2003 to 29.2% in 2007. Patients with private insurance were 10 times more likely to undergo reconstruction than patients with Medi-Cal insurance (OR 9.95, 95% CI 8.46–11.70). African American patients were less likely (OR 0.58, 95% CI 0.46–0.73) and Asian patients one-third as likely (OR 0.37, 95% CI 0.29–0.47) to undergo reconstruction as Caucasians patients Most reconstructive procedures were performed at teaching hospitals and designated cancer centers.

Conclusions.—Although the rate of postmastectomy reconstruction is increasing, only a minority of patients undergo reconstruction. Age, race, type of insurance, and type of hospital appear to be significant factors limiting the use of reconstruction.

▶ The increasing use of breast conservation surgery has clearly reduced the numbers of patients who might be candidates for breast reconstruction. Yet for patients who have undergone a therapeutic or prophylactic mastectomy, it has been clearly demonstrated, for many years, that breast reconstruction after mastectomy is safe and usually effective, does not contribute to the incidence of tumor recurrence or negatively affect survival, and does provide patients with real and perceived psychological and physical benefit. However, as in many other studies,[1,2] the actual rate of reconstruction, although increasing annually, still remains low. The authors of this study point to a number of variables that contribute to this, including socioeconomic factors, age of the patient, type of insurance, type of hospital, and others. It is true that the reasons patients do not undergo breast reconstruction are varied and likely complex, but missing from this study, largely because of the data source (California Office of Statewide

Health Planning and Development), are the percentage of patients who actually had informed consent—that is, how many actually knew about the reconstructive options and had an opportunity to make an informed choice? It is not likely that those who are unaware of the possibility of reconstructive surgery would opt to undergo such surgery.

S. H. Miller, MD

References

1. Chen JY, Malin J, Ganz PA, et al. Variation in physician-patient discussion of breast reconstruction. *J Gen Intern Med*. 2009;24:99-104.
2. Morrow M, Mujahid M, Lantz PM, et al. Correlates of breast reconstruction: results from a population-based study. *Cancer*. 2005;104:2340-2346.

The use of imaging in patients post breast reconstruction
Sim YT, Litherland JC (Glasgow Royal Infirmary, UK)
Clin Radiol 67:128-133, 2012

Aim.—To evaluate the usefulness of mammographic surveillance for asymptomatic patients and as a problem-solving tool in symptomatic patients with reconstructed breasts.

Materials and Methods.—The imaging records over 4 years identified 227 patients with a history of breast reconstruction post-mastectomy due to cancer. Clinical and imaging records were reviewed to evaluate the use of imaging in the follow-up management of these patients.

Results.—Records showed that 116 (51%) of the patients identified underwent surveillance mammography of the reconstructed breast, in which one recurrent cancer was detected in an autologous tissue flap reconstruction (0.86% detection rate of non-palpable recurrent cancer), with a recall rate of 4%. One other patient had interval recurrence diagnosed following presentation with pain. Mammography of the contralateral breast only was performed in 111 patients. Fifty-four patients (24%) presented on 78 occasions with symptoms relating to the breast reconstructions, most commonly lump or swelling. Half of these patient episodes subsequently found no significant abnormality, and a further 29% had fat necrosis revealed on imaging. Four recurrent cancers were diagnosed.

Conclusion.—There is insufficient evidence for recommending routine surveillance mammography for non-palpable recurrent cancer in the reconstructed breasts. Ultrasound and mammography are useful imaging techniques in the assessment of reconstructed breasts in the symptomatic setting. Fat necrosis is the most common benign finding on mammograms of reconstructed breasts, both in the surveillance and symptomatic groups.

▶ The crux of the issue, in my view, is that plastic surgeons who perform reconstructive breast surgery must continue to be an integral part of the team following patients who have undergone mastectomy and reconstruction. While I agree with the suggestion that routine surveillance mammography of asymptomatic reconstructed breast is probably "overkill," resulting in added costs with little benefit, I do believe its use is warranted in symptomatic patients but especially in those patients who have undergone partial mastectomy or breast conservation mastectomy. I also believe that a worthwhile multidisciplinary project, among interested specialists, to develop best practices for following patients who have had a mastectomy and reconstruction is long overdo.

S. H. Miller, MD

Tamoxifen Increases the Risk of Microvascular Flap Complications in Patients Undergoing Microvascular Breast Reconstruction
Kelley BP, Valero V, Yi M, et al (The Univ of Texas M. D. Anderson Cancer Ctr, Houston)
Plast Reconstr Surg 129:305-314, 2012

Background.—Tamoxifen citrate (tamoxifen) has been associated with increased rates of thromboembolic events, prompting concerns that it may increase the risk of complications after microvascular breast reconstruction. Some centers have implemented protocols to temporarily stop tamoxifen before microvascular breast reconstruction. The authors sought to determine whether this practice is warranted.

Methods.—A total of 670 patients underwent delayed microsurgical breast reconstruction at the authors' institution between January of 2000 and April of 2010. Rates of microvascular flap complications and pulmonary emboli were retrospectively compared between patients who were and were not receiving tamoxifen at the time of reconstruction.

Results.—A total of 205 patients received tamoxifen within 28 days before reconstruction (these patients were considered to be receiving tamoxifen at reconstruction); 465 patients did not. Those who received tamoxifen were significantly younger ($p < 0.0001$) and thinner ($p = 0.0025$), with less cardiovascular morbidity ($p = 0.04$) and shorter durations of operations ($p = 0.05$). Despite fewer comorbidities, microvascular flap complications were significantly more common among tamoxifen patients (21.5 versus 15 percent; $p = 0.04$). They had 1.7 times the risk of complications ($p = 0.015$) and 1.8 times the risk of follow-up complications ($p = 0.03$) than no-tamoxifen patients. In the tamoxifen group, cardiovascular comorbidities significantly increased the risk of flap complications ($p = 0.002$). Tamoxifen patients had a significantly increased rate of immediate total flap loss ($p = 0.041$) and a lower rate of flap salvage ($p = 0.023$). Tamoxifen did not appear to increase the risk of pulmonary embolus during or after delayed microvascular breast reconstruction.

Conclusions.—Tamoxifen may increase the risk of microvascular flap complications. Surgeons should consider temporarily stopping the drug 28 days before microsurgical breast reconstruction.

Clinical Question/Level of Evidence.—Risk, II.

▶ This study raises a red flag and several important questions regarding the timing of the use of tamoxifen in patients scheduled to undergo delayed microvascular breast reconstruction. The findings show that overall flap complications, total flap loss, and lower flap salvage rate were more frequent in patients on tamoxifen. But caution needs to be exercised, as this is a retrospective study with small groups of patients and even smaller numbers of complications upon which to base conclusions. For example, the average ages of the patients on tamoxifen versus those not on tamoxifen were statistically younger. Do we know whether the ages of the patients on tamoxifen vary, and did the older patients have fewer complications than did their younger counterparts? Why did the incidence of pulmonary embolism not differ between the tamoxifen and nontamoxifen groups? Why did the group undergoing reconstruction with donor tissue from areas other than the abdomen have a greater incidence of microvascular complications? Is there evidence that stopping tamoxifen for 28 days is really necessary as opposed to 7 or 14 days?

S. H. Miller, MD

Accurate Assessment of Breast Volume: A Study Comparing the Volumetric Gold Standard (Direct Water Displacement Measurement of Mastectomy Specimen) With a 3D Laser Scanning Technique
Yip JM, Mouratova N, Jeffery RM, et al (Flinders Med Centre, South Australia; Flinders Univ, South Australia; et al)
Ann Plast Surg 68:135-141, 2012

Preoperative assessment of breast volume could contribute significantly to the planning of breast-related procedures. The availability of 3D scanning technology provides us with an innovative method for doing this. We performed this study to compare measurements by this technology with breast volume measurement by water displacement. A total of 30 patients undergoing 39 mastectomies were recruited from our center. The volume of each patient's breast(s) was determined with a preoperative 3D laser scan. The volume of the mastectomy specimen was then measured in the operating theater by water displacement. There was a strong linear association between breast volumes measured using the 2 different methods when using a Pearson correlation ($r = 0.95$, $P < 0.001$). The mastectomy mean volume was defined by the equation: mastectomy mean volume = (scan mean volume × 1.03) −70.6. This close correlation validates the Cyberware WBX Scanner as a tool for assessment of breast volume (Figs 1-3).

▶ Potentially, this is an interesting aid to "re-creating" a breast, similar in size, to the one that has been removed during the course of treatment for breast cancer (Figs 1, 2, and 3). Several issues remain to be clarified before accepting the use of this modality as a standard. I appreciated the authors' attempt to

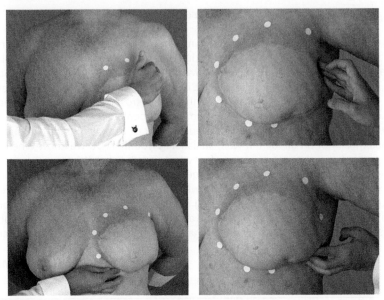

FIGURE 1.—Determination of the breast borders by palpation, and placement of landmarking stickers. (Reprinted from Yip JM, Mouratova N, Jeffery RM, et al. Accurate assessment of breast volume: a study comparing the volumetric gold standard (direct water displacement measurement of mastectomy specimen) with a 3D laser scanning technique. *Ann Plast Surg*. 2012;68:135-141, with permission from Lippincott Williams & Wilkins.)

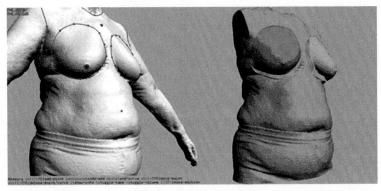

FIGURE 2.—Utilizing CySlice (Cyberware) to section the breast portion of the scan from the torso for volume analysis. (Reprinted from Yip JM, Mouratova N, Jeffery RM, et al. Accurate assessment of breast volume: a study comparing the volumetric gold standard (direct water displacement measurement of mastectomy specimen) with a 3D laser scanning technique. *Ann Plast Surg*. 2012;68:135-141, with permission from Lippincott Williams & Wilkins.)

individualize the size and extent of the breast tissue by direct palpation, but I am unsure of the interrater reliability of this method. I am also uncertain of the accuracy of this technique in both larger breasts and ptotic breasts. Finally, the authors have not given an indication of the costs involved in using this

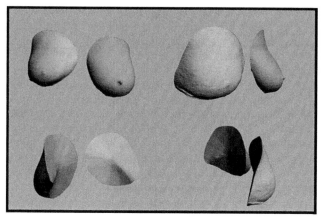

FIGURE 3.—The concavity of the posterior surface of the breast is taken into account by the scanner when sectioning the breast away from the torso. (Reprinted from Yip JM, Mouratova N, Jeffery RM, et al. Accurate assessment of breast volume: a study comparing the volumetric gold standard (direct water displacement measurement of mastectomy specimen) with a 3D laser scanning technique. *Ann Plast Surg*. 2012;68:135-141, with permission from Lippincott Williams & Wilkins.)

technique and whether they are justified over the gold standard water displacement methods. It will be interesting to see follow-up studies to address some of these issues.

S. H. Miller, MD

A Head-to-Head Comparison of Quality of Life and Aesthetic Outcomes following Immediate, Staged-Immediate, and Delayed Oncoplastic Reduction Mammaplasty

Patel KM, Hannan CM, Gatti ME, et al (Georgetown Univ Hosp, Washington, DC)
Plast Reconstr Surg 127:2167-2175, 2011

Background.—Oncoplastic reduction mammaplasty offers patients breast conservation with the added benefit of functional improvement in symptoms related to macromastia. The reduction can be performed in the immediate setting with the lumpectomy, in a staged-immediate fashion after final pathology has been confirmed or in a delayed fashion after completion of both lumpectomy and radiation. This study compared quality of life and aesthetic outcomes for these different cohorts.

Methods.—A retrospective review was carried out on 16 consecutive patients who had oncoplastic reduction mammaplasty by the senior author (M.Y.N.) between 2003 and 2009. Demographics, oncologic treatment and timing, and reduction techniques were recorded. Patients were asked to complete a questionnaire to assess quality of life and satisfaction. Preoperative and postoperative photographs were evaluated by 15 reviewers.

Results.—Over a 7-year period, five patients had immediate, six had staged-immediate, and five had delayed reduction mammaplasty. Mean patient age was 52.5 years, and mean body mass index was 31.5. The average timing of reduction was 0, 49, and 734 days for the three groups. Positive margins occurred in two patients, leading to completion mastectomy. In addition, one patient in the staged-immediate group had a recurrence that led to completion mastectomy. Complications occurred in seven (44 percent) of 16 patients. Questionnaire response was 75 percent (12 of 16), showing positive scores in all groups but no statistical significance. Objective aesthetic evaluation also revealed significant improvements within groups comparing various preoperative to postoperative parameters. Importantly, aesthetic scores for the delayed group were consistently lower across all aspects but did not reach significance.

Conclusion.—Oncoplastic reduction mammaplasty can be safe and effective in carefully selected patients in the immediate, staged-immediate, and delayed settings.

▶ This study reconfirms the value of oncoplastic reduction mammaplasty, but still leaves open some questions regarding the appropriate timing of the procedure—immediate, staged-immediate, or delayed. There is clearly great benefit in offering patients "2-for-1" therapy—the opportunity to treat their breast cancer and alleviate their symptoms of macromastia in a single operation. Studies have repeatedly confirmed the oncologic effectiveness of lumpectomy + reduction + radiation. This study gives us some hints of information that can help make the judgment about timing. Unfortunately, the numbers of patients in the study do not allow the translation of these hints into statistically significant conclusions. There is value in recognizing, for example, that the chances of having positive margins after staged-immediate surgery were lower than those after immediate surgery and that the lowest scores for aesthetic appearance were recorded after delayed treatment. A larger series might allow these interesting observations to reach statistical significance. Until then, these findings can suggest treatment, but not definitively direct it.

R. L. Ruberg, MD

Reconstructive Outcomes in Patients Undergoing Contralateral Prophylactic Mastectomy
Crosby MA, Garvey PB, Selber JC, et al (The Univ of Texas MD Anderson Cancer Ctr, Houston; The Johns Hopkins Hosp, Baltimore, MD)
Plast Reconstr Surg 128:1025-1033, 2011

Background.—As the rate of contralateral prophylactic mastectomy in breast cancer patients increases, more women are seeking immediate bilateral breast reconstruction. The authors evaluated complication rates in the index and prophylactic breasts in patients undergoing bilateral immediate reconstruction.

Methods.—The authors retrospectively reviewed the outcomes of all consecutive patients undergoing immediate postmastectomy bilateral reconstruction for an index breast cancer combined with a contralateral prophylactic mastectomy between 2005 and 2010. Patient, tumor, reconstruction, and outcome characteristics were compared between the index and prophylactic breasts in the same patient. Patients were classified by reconstruction method: implant, abdominal flap, or latissimus dorsi flap/implant. Regression models evaluated patient and reconstruction characteristics for potential predictive or protective associations with postoperative complications.

Results.—Of 497 patients included, 334 (67.2 percent) underwent implant reconstruction, 142 (28.6 percent) had abdominal flap reconstruction, and 21 (4.2 percent) had latissimus dorsi flap/implant reconstruction. Index reconstructions had a complication rate (22.5 percent) equivalent to that of contralateral prophylactic mastectomy reconstructions (19.1 percent; $p = 0.090$). Overall, 101 patients (20.3 percent) developed a complication in one reconstructed breast, and 53 (10.7 percent) developed complications in both breasts. Of the 154 patients who developed complications, 42 (27.3 percent) developed a complication in the prophylactic breast.

Conclusions.—Immediate index and contralateral prophylactic breast reconstructions appear to have equivalent outcomes, both overall and across reconstruction classifications. Together, patients, reconstructive surgeons, and extirpative surgeons should carefully consider the oncologic benefits of a contralateral prophylactic mastectomy in light of the risk of increased surgical morbidity of this type of mastectomy and reconstruction.

▶ This is an important, albeit retrospective, study that must be read carefully. At the outset, one must question whether the authors really meant to say that "patients, reconstructive and extirpative surgeons should carefully consider the oncologic benefits of a prophylactic mastectomy in light of the increased surgical morbidity of this type of mastectomy and reconstruction." In fact, the authors did not study the oncologic benefits of prophylactic mastectomy at all, but the risks of immediate reconstruction after prophylactic and therapeutic mastectomy. Roughly 20% of the patients had complications as a result of the combined extirpative and reconstructive procedures regardless of whether the procedure was therapeutic or prophylactic or the type of reconstruction. Would the complication rates have been the same if the reconstruction had been delayed in both the extirpative and prophylactic groups? While patients tend to be happier if extirpation and reconstruction are performed in a single sitting, they are less pleased when the latter results in complications.

S. H. Miller, MD

Tissue-Engineered Breast Reconstruction: Bridging the Gap Toward Large-Volume Tissue Engineering in Humans

Findlay MW, Dolderer JH, Trost N, et al (O'Brien Institute, Melbourne, Australia; St Vincent's Hosp Melbourne, Australia; Univ of Melbourne, Victoria, Australia)
Plast Reconstr Surg 128:1206-1215, 2011

Background.—Use of autologous tissue is ideal in breast reconstruction; however, insufficient donor tissue and surgical and donor-site morbidity all limit its use. Tissue engineering could provide replacement tissue, but only if vascularization of large tissue volumes is achievable. The authors sought to upscale their small-animal adipose tissue-engineering models to produce large volumes of tissue in a large animal (i.e., pig).

Methods.—Bilateral large-volume (78.5 ml) chambers were inserted subcutaneously in the groin enclosing a fat flap (5 ml) based on the superficial circumflex iliac pedicle for 6 ($n = 4$), 12 ($n = 1$), and 22 weeks ($n = 2$).

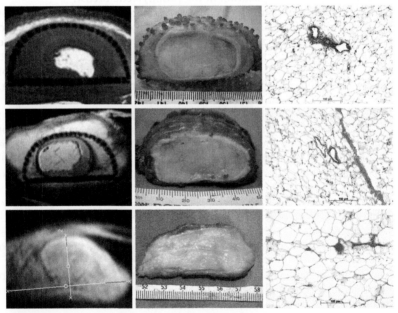

FIGURE 3.—Chamber specimens 6 (*above*), 12 (*center*), and 22 (*below*) weeks after insertion showing (*left to right*) magnetic resonance imaging scan, cut surface of corresponding whole specimen, and central histologic image. Cross-sectional area of adipose tissue increases with increasing time in vivo, analyzed by magnetic resonance imaging and confirmed macroscopically (*above, center,* and *below*). Note capsule of fibrovascular tissue immediately adjacent to the polycarbonate chamber. The poly (L-lactide-co-glycolide) scaffold between the capsule and central fat shows expansion in volume during its breakdown from 6 to 12 weeks, with very little remaining by 22 weeks. Adipose tissue growth between 6 and 12 weeks is not associated with significant cell hypertrophy, but regional cell hypertrophy is evident by 22 weeks when compared with fat flap tissue at chamber insertion. (Reprinted from Findlay MW, Dolderer JH, Trost N, et al. Tissue-engineered breast reconstruction: bridging the gap toward large-volume tissue engineering in humans. *Plast Reconstr Surg.* 2011;128:1206-1215, with permission from the American Society of Plastic Surgeons.)

Right chambers included a poly (L-lactide-co-glycolide) sponge. Other pedicle configurations, including a vascular pedicle alone ($n = 2$) or in combination with muscle ($n = 2$) or a free fat graft ($n = 2$), were investigated in preliminary studies. Serial assessment of tissue growth and vascularization by magnetic resonance imaging was undertaken during growth and correlated with quantitative histomorphometry at chamber removal.

Results.—All chambers filled with new tissue by 6 weeks, vascularized by the arteriovenous pedicle. In the fat flap chambers, the initial 5 ml of fat expanded to 25.9 ± 2.4, 39.4 ± 3.9, and 56.5 ml (by magnetic resonance imaging) at 6, 12, and 22 weeks, respectively. Adipose tissue volume was maintained up to 22 weeks after chamber removal ($n = 2$), including one where the specimen was transferred on its pedicle to an adjacent submammary pocket.

Conclusion.—The first clinically relevant volumes of tissue for in situ and remote breast reconstruction have been formed with implications for scaling of existing tissue-engineering models into human trials (Fig 3).

▶ This is a fascinating study in pigs. The translation of small animal success in growing fat into success with large animals is terrific. Whether this work can be replicated with larger numbers of animals and whether the specific factors that result in fat generation can be isolated remain to be documented. Of course, the drawbacks, when translating this model to humans, are the need to grow the fat over time, the costs involved, the need to use, at least temporarily, a donor area as a site for growing the fat and to sacrifice vasculature in the donor area, and longer-term follow-up to document that the fat transplanted maintains it size and shape. Ultimately, how will the risks, costs, and benefits of this technique match up with the current methods of breast reconstruction (Fig 3)?

S. H. Miller, MD

Body Lift Perforator Flap Breast Reconstruction: A Review of 100 Flaps in 25 Cases

DellaCroce FJ, Sullivan SK, Trahan C, et al (Ctr for Restorative Breast Surgery, New Orleans, LA)
Plast Reconstr Surg 129:551-561, 2012

Background.—Advances in autologous breast reconstruction continue to mount and have been fueled most substantially with refinement of perforator flap techniques.

Methods.—For patients with a desire for autogenous breast reconstruction and insufficient abdominal fat for conventional abdominal flaps, secondary options such as gluteal perforator flaps or latissimus flaps are usually considered. Patients who also have insufficient soft tissue in the gluteal donor site and preference to avoid an implant, present a vexing problem. The authors describe an option that allows for incorporation of four independent perforator flaps for bilateral breast reconstruction when individual donor sites are too thin to provide necessary volume. The authors

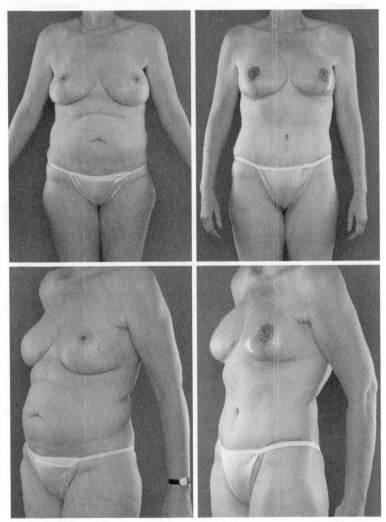

FIGURE 9.—Preoperative *(left)* and postoperative*(right)*views of a patient who underwent bilateral mastectomy with immediate body lift perforator flap breast reconstruction. Mastectomy weights were 620 and 800 g, and the combined weight of two DIEP/GAP flaps in each associated breast was 865 and 765 g. Radiated skin envelope on left with resultant mild peripheral contour constriction. (Reprinted from DellaCroce FJ, Sullivan SK, Trahan C, et al. Body lift perforator flap breast reconstruction: a review of 100 flaps in 25 cases. *Plast Reconstr Surg.* 2012;129:551-561, with permission from the American Society of Plastic Surgeons.)

present their experience with this technique in 25 patients with 100 individual flaps over 5 years.

Results.—The body lift perforator flap technique, using a layered deep inferior epigastric perforator/gluteal perforator flap combination for each breast, was performed in this patient set with high success rates and quality

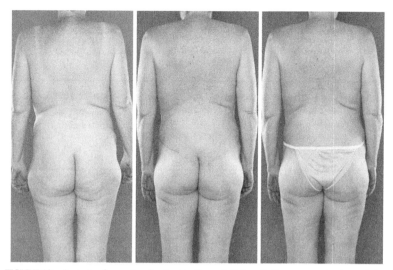

FIGURE 10.—Posterior donor site of patient in Figure 9. Before (*left*), postoperative (*center*) demonstrating preserved gluteal aesthetic, and easily hidden scarline placement (*right*). (Reprinted from DellaCroce FJ, Sullivan SK, Trahan C, et al. Body lift perforator flap breast reconstruction: a review of 100 flaps in 25 cases. *Plast Reconstr Surg.* 2012;129:551-561, with permission from the American Society of Plastic Surgeons.)

aesthetic outcomes over several years. Patient satisfaction was high among the studied population.

Conclusions.—The body lift perforator flap breast reconstruction technique can be a reliable, safe, but technically demanding solution for patients seeking autogenous breast reconstruction with otherwise inadequate individual fatty donor sites. This sophisticated procedure overcomes a limitation of autogenous breast reconstruction for these patients that otherwise results in a breast with poor projection and overall volume insufficiency. The harvest of truncal fat with a circumferential body lift design gives the potential added benefit of improved body contour as a complement to this powerful breast reconstructive technique.

Clinical Question/Level of Evidence.—Therapeutic, IV (Figs 9 and 10).

▶ This is an interesting surgical tour de force. Several questions can be posed. Is there a good method by which the surgeon can judge which patients have inadequate fatty donor sites and thus how much tissue is actually required for autologous reconstruction? When faced with paucity of soft tissue, using a deep inferior epigastric perforator/superficial inferior epigastric artery or gluteal artery perforator (GAP) flap, do the authors consider using a standard split pedicled a deepithelialized transverse rectus abdominis myocutaneous flap (Fig 9)? Would an inferior GAP flap in older patients better improve the cosmetic appearance of the buttock region these patients (Fig 10)? Overall, the results shown are quite good, but are they typical? The assessment of the postoperative results is limited by a relatively poor follow-up, 36%, and we are not told when this follow-up occurred.

S. H. Miller, MD

Immediate Free Flap Reconstruction for Advanced-Stage Breast Cancer: Is It Safe?
Crisera CA, Chang EI, Da Lio AL, et al (Univ of California, Los Angeles; Memorial Sloan-Kettering Cancer Ctr, NY)
Plast Reconstr Surg 128:32-41, 2011

Background.—Numerous studies have demonstrated that immediate breast reconstruction following mastectomy is associated with improvements in quality of life and body image. However, immediate breast reconstruction for advanced-stage breast cancer remains controversial. This study evaluates its safety in patients with advanced-stage breast cancer.

Methods.—Over a 10-year period, patients diagnosed with stage IIB or greater breast cancer treated with mastectomy followed by immediate breast reconstruction were identified and analyzed. Complication rates and reconstructive aesthetics were determined.

Results.—One hundred seventy patients were identified who underwent 157 unilateral and 13 bilateral reconstructions (183 flaps) predominantly by means of free transverse rectus abdominis musculocutaneous flaps ($n = 162$). The average age was 47 years and the average hospital stay was 5.1 days. There were 15 major complications (8.8 percent), but adjuvant postoperative therapy was delayed in only eight patients (4.7 percent), with the maximum delay lasting 3 weeks in one patient. Although some degree of flap shrinkage was noted in 30 percent of patients treated with postoperative radiotherapy, only 10 percent of patients experienced severe breast distortion. Importantly, the overall cosmetic outcome in patients who underwent postoperative irradiation was comparable to that of those who did not.

Conclusions.—The authors have shown that immediate breast reconstruction in the setting of advanced-stage breast cancer is safe and well tolerated by patients, and is not associated with significant delays in adjuvant therapy. These findings make a strong argument for immediate reconstruction regardless of cancer stage. The authors found the changes caused by radiation to the reconstructed breast to be less significant than previously reported and readily addressed to complete an ultimate reconstruction that is aesthetically acceptable to both surgeon and patient.

Clinical Question/Level of Evidence.—Therapeutic, IV.

▶ This article presents some findings regarding immediate breast reconstruction that are consistent with previous studies and some findings that are not. The consistent findings focus principally on the safety and effectiveness of immediate reconstruction in patients with advanced breast cancer. In part, this study is valuable because it reaffirms previous findings about complication rates in these patients but in a series that is more than twice as large as in previous studies.

Once again, the study shows that the complication rates for immediate free tissue transfer for advance-stage breast cancer are no different than those seen in treatment for earlier-stage patients. What differs from many previous reports is the finding that only a small percentage of patients experienced significant postradiation deformity of the reconstructed breast. This finding does not specifically relate to the "safety" of immediate reconstruction in the advanced-stage patients, only to the ultimate cosmetic result. But because of the conflict with some previous reports, this particular aspect of this report warrants further investigation.

R. L. Ruberg, MD

Breast Reconstruction Using the Lateral Femoral Circumflex Artery Perforator Flap

Kind GM, Foster RD (California-Pacific Med Ctr, San Francisco; Univ of California—San Francisco)
J Reconstr Microsurg 27:427-431, 2011

The development of microsurgical breast reconstruction has resulted in not only the lower abdomen as a source of donor site tissue but also interest in alternative donor sites. These have included perforator-based flaps at the sites of previously described myocutaneous flaps (e.g., superior or inferior gluteal arteries) and the use of myocutaneous flaps not previously used for breast reconstruction (e.g., gracilis or transverse upper gracilis). We present our experience with a unique form of the tensor fascia lata flap and describe the first reported use of the lateral femoral circumflex artery (LFCA) perforator flap for breast reconstruction. A patient with minimal abdominal fat but lipodystrophy of the upper lateral thighs presented for breast reconstruction. Perforator flaps based on the lateral femoral circumflex vessels were designed. The LFCA perforator flap from one side was successfully used for breast reconstruction. The flap on the contralateral side did not have a suitable perforator. The LFCA perforator flap offers another option for women seeking autogenous breast reconstruction. Advances in preoperative imaging will likely make this a more reliable option (Fig 1).

▶ Some plastic surgeons may wonder about the choice of autologous reconstruction in this case report, as a 1- or 2-stage prosthetic reconstruction with nipple-sparing mastectomies could have provided an excellent result without the additional scars that would need to be hidden beneath clothing and be visible in a swimsuit. Given this case example, with the desire to harvest upper lateral thigh skin and fat for an autologous reconstruction, the potential utility for preoperative perforator angiography via computed tomography or magnetic resonance imaging is demonstrated. With the distribution of her fat in the upper saddlebag area (Fig 1), it is conceivable that the main blood supply could arise from an anterior (lateral circumflex femoral) or posterior (inferior gluteal artery) source. Preoperative imaging may have been able to elucidate a prominent perforator and subsequent source vessel and then allow for optimal skin paddle design.

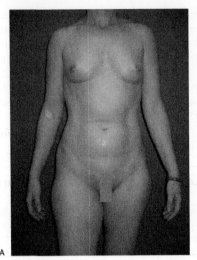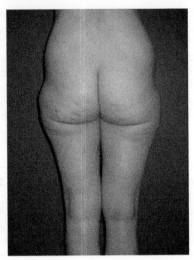

A B

FIGURE 1.—Preoperative views of a 39-year-old woman with high risk of breast cancer. (A) Front view; (B) Back view. (Reprinted from Kind GM, Foster RD. Breast reconstruction using the lateral femoral circumflex artery perforator flap. *J Reconstr Microsurg.* 2011;27:427-431, with permission from Thieme Medical Publishers, Inc.)

Regardless, this case study reminds us that if there is an adequate perforator with adequate fat, it can be harvested for a breast reconstruction.

J. Boehmler, MD

Deep Femoral Artery Perforator Flap: A New Perforator Flap for Breast Reconstruction

Schneider LF, Vasile JV, Levine JL, et al (New York Univ Langone Med Ctr; Ctr for Microsurgical Breast Reconstruction, NY)
J Reconstr Microsurg 27:531-536, 2011

We present the deep femoral artery perforator (DFAP) flap, a new perforator flap for breast reconstruction, with a detailed description of operative technique and four clinical examples. The DFAP flap allows harvest of tissue from the lower buttock and lateral thigh with similar territory to an in-the-crease inferior gluteal artery perforator (IGAP) flap but based on a different perforator. When present, the DFAP is the largest vessel supplying this territory and is often septocutaneous, facilitating dissection when compared with the IGAP flap. We used preoperative imaging with magnetic resonance angiography to assist in accurate flap planning which also permitted precise determination of perforator origin. In patients with either a contraindication to abdominal wall-based perforator flaps or weight

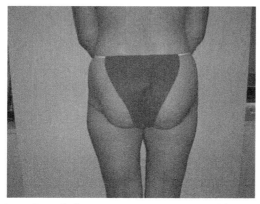

FIGURE 8.—Postoperative results for Case 4, posterior view. (Reprinted from Schneider LF, Vasile JV, Levine JL, et al. Deep femoral artery perforator flap: a new perforator flap for breast reconstruction. *J Reconstr Microsurg.* 2011;27:531-536, with permission from Thieme Medical Publishers, Inc.)

distribution below the waist, the DFAP flap provides an alternative to the IGAP flap with an excellent pedicle and a favorable location on the lateral thigh (Fig 8).

▶ This refinement of a lower buttock, upper thigh flap seems to be a worthwhile addition to the armamentarium of the microvascular reconstructive breast surgeon. Its appeal, in this limited series, is the uniformity of the donor tissue thickness, especially in thin patients, and the lateral position of the donor tissue when compared with the inferior gluteal artery perforator flap. The use of preoperative magnetic resonance angiography is important in planning the procedure.

S. H. Miller, MD

Trials and Tribulations with the Inferior Gluteal Artery Perforator Flap in Autologous Breast Reconstruction

Mirzabeigi MN, Au A, Jandali S, et al (Univ of Pennsylvania, Philadelphia)
Plast Reconstr Surg 128:614e-624e, 2011

Background.—Perforator free flaps from the buttock serve as an alternative to abdominally based flaps in autologous breast reconstruction. Microsurgeons often opt to harvest tissue from the gluteal donor site because of a lack of abdominal volume and/or quality. The authors examined the experience of a single surgeon with the inferior gluteal artery perforator (IGAP) flap and provide a quantitative outcomes comparison with the deep inferior epigastric perforator (DIEP) flap.

Methods.—A retrospective review was performed of patients who underwent IGAP flap surgery for autologous breast reconstruction from August of 2005 to October of 2010 performed by a single surgeon (J.M.S.).

Results.—Thirty-one inferior gluteal artery perforator flaps were performed on 24 patients. Mean follow-up time was 24.4 months (range, 6

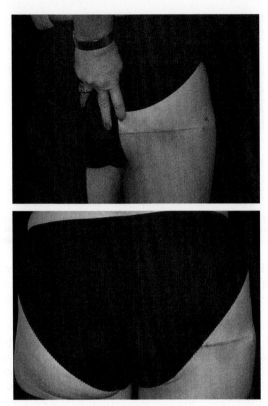

FIGURE 2.—*(Above)* The donor site can be largely concealed through most types of undergarments or swimwear; however, postoperative asymmetry *(below)* is common, which prompts a donor-site revision in many patients. (Reprinted from Mirzabeigi MN, Au A, Jandali S, et al. Trials and tribulations with the inferior gluteal artery perforator flap in autologous breast reconstruction. *Plast Reconstr Surg.* 2011;128:614e-624e, with permission from the American Society of Plastic Surgeons.)

to 65 months). The total flap loss rate was 6.5 percent, and the take-back rate was 13 percent (salvage rate, 75 percent). Vascular complication rates were as follows: intraoperative arterial thrombosis, 13 percent; intraoperative venous thrombosis, 3 percent; delayed arterial thrombosis, 3 percent; and delayed venous thrombosis, 13 percent. Nineteen percent of patients had sensory complaints at the donor site that persisted beyond 3 months postoperatively. In comparison to the DIEP flap, IGAP flaps had a higher rate of intraoperative arterial thrombosis (13 percent versus 2.6 percent, $p = 0.024$) and delayed venous thrombosis (13 percent versus 1.5 percent, $p = 0.008$).

Conclusions.—Review of the IGAP flap reveals some shortcomings of this flap even in the hands of an experienced microsurgeon. Surgeons should be aware of the difficulties and limitations when choosing this flap for reconstruction (Fig 2).

▶ This is a worthwhile and instructive contribution to the literature of autologous breast reconstruction primarily because it documents the difficulties that can befall even the most experienced microsurgical team. Whether the distinctions made, in this report, between the authors' experiences with the deep inferior epigastric perforator (DIEP) flap and the inferior gluteal artery perforator (IGAP) flap are real, because the indications for use of the IGAP flap are clearly different, the high incidence of vascular complications, especially those related to late venous thrombosis are problematic; one wonders whether better control of the disparity in venous size between donor and recipient vessel will adequately address this problem. Equally disconcerting is the relatively high incidence of volume deficiency and projection requiring further augmentation of the reconstructed breast as well as the rather significant deformity at the donor site (Fig 2). The latter seems to be less of an issue with the lateralization of the gluteal buttock using the deep femoral artery perforator (DFAP).[1] The DFAP may also better overcome the disparity between the donor and recipient veins noted in the authors' experience with the IGAP flap.

S. H. Miller, MD

Reference

1. Schneider LF, Vasile JV, Levine JL, Allen RJ. Deep femoral artery perforator flap: a new perforator flap for breast reconstruction. *J Reconstr Microsurg.* 2011;27: 531-536.

Modifications to Extend the Transverse Upper Gracilis Flap in Breast Reconstruction: Clinical Series and Results
Saint-Cyr M, Wong C, Oni G, et al (Univ of Texas Southwestern Med Ctr, Dallas; Univ of Lyon, France)
Plast Reconstr Surg 129:24e-36e, 2012

Background.—The transverse myocutaneous gracilis flap has traditionally been used to reconstruct smaller breasts. The authors have been performing autologous breast reconstruction utilizing the flap with two types of modifications to increase flap volume: an extended and a vertical extended flap. In this article, they discuss the different operative techniques and present a clinical series of both flap types.

Methods.—A retrospective review of all patients undergoing either flap modification under the senior author (M.S.-C.) was performed. Data collated included pedicle artery and vein diameters, flap weight, and patient complications.

Results.—Twenty-four transverse myocutaneous gracilis flaps were performed: 12 extended (seven patients) and 12 vertical flaps (six patients). The vertical group trended to have greater flap weights than the extended

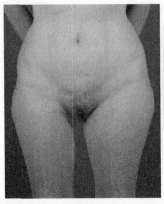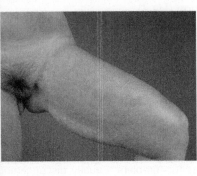

FIGURE 13.—(*Left*) Postoperative view of donor site after1 year after unilateral breast reconstruction with an extended flap. Limiting the incision anteriorly and keeping it close to the inguinal crease will help hide the final scar. (*Right*) Final donor-site appearance at 6 months after a vertical flap (trilobe) harvest. (Reprinted from Saint-Cyr M, Wong C, Oni G, et al. Modifications to extend the transverse upper gracilis flap in breast reconstruction: clinical series and results. *Plast Reconstr Surg.* 2012;129:24e-36e, with permission from the American Society of Plastic Surgeons.)

group. Mean flap weight was 385.75 g (range, 181 to 750 g) for the extended group and 469.75 g (range, 380 to 605 g) for the vertical group ($p = 0.06$). Mean arterial diameter of the medial circumflex artery was 1.9 mm (range, 1.5 to 2.0 mm), mean venous diameter was 2.4 mm (range, 2.0 to 3.5 mm), and mean pedicle length was 6.8 cm (range, 6.0 to 7.0 cm). All donor sites were closed primarily. Complications included seroma ($n = 1$), wound dehiscence ($n = 2$), and partial flap loss ($n = 2$).

Conclusions.—Modifications of the transverse myocutaneous gracilis flap increase flap volume and can be useful in patients who do not wish to have abdomen, buttock, or back scars. Donor-site scars can be concealed, and patients have the added benefit of a thigh lift. Complications are comparable to those found with other reconstructive options.

Clinical Question/Level of Evidence.—Therapeutic, III (Fig 13).

▶ The search continues for more and, in some instances, better and safer sites for alternative flaps for breast reconstruction. The authors have modified the transverse upper gracilis flap for breast reconstruction to increase its utility for reconstructing moderately large breasts.[1] Of the 24 flaps created in 13 patients, several photos demonstrating the appearance of postoperative donor site are provided, but most of the photos are not good representations of the breast reconstruction achieved. Further, the incidence of complications—fat necrosis in 17% of the flaps and flap necrosis in 13%—seems a bit high, especially when these complications are likely related to the need to increase the amount of fat incorporated in these flaps, a goal achievable by implanting a smaller and safer flap augmented by fat grafting. Additionally, the patient shown in Fig 13 might have been a better candidate for a deep femoral artery perforator flap.[2] Nonetheless, the gracilis flap remains a useful addition to the armamentarium of the reconstructive breast surgeon.

S. H. Miller, MD

References

1. Fattah A, Figus A, Mathur B. The transverse myocutaneous gracilis flap: technical refinements. *J Plast Reconstr Aesthet Surg.* 2010;63:305-313.
2. Schneider LF, Vasile JV, Levine JL, Allen RJ. Deep femoral artery perforator flap: a new perforator flap for breast reconstruction. *J Reconstr Microsurg.* 2011;27: 531-536.

The Low Transverse Extended Latissimus Dorsi Flap Based on Fat Compartments of the Back for Breast Reconstruction: Anatomical Study and Clinical Results

Bailey SH, Saint-Cyr M, Oni G, et al (Univ of Texas Southwestern Med Ctr at Dallas; Univ of Lyon, France)
Plast Reconstr Surg 128:382e-394e, 2011

Background.—Despite many modifications to the extended latissimus dorsi flap, its use in autologous breast reconstruction remains limited because of insufficient volume and donor-site morbidity. Through a detailed analysis of the deposition of back fat, this study describes a low transverse extended latissimus dorsi flap harvest technique that increases flap volumes and improves donor-site aesthetics.

Methods.—Eight fresh cadaver hemibacks were used to identify the anatomical location of the fat compartments. Correlation between the fat compartments and the fat folds was made using photographic analysis of 216 patients. Retrospective case note review was conducted of all patients

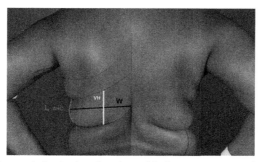

FIGURE 1.—Photograph showing how the volume of the fat compartments can be estimated with the formula $L_{arc} \times (w) \times 1/2\, vh$, where L_{arc} is the arc length of the fat compartment, w is the width of the compartment from the spinous process to the lateral skin edge on the posterior axillary line of the fat folds, and vh is the vertical height of the compartment. (Reprinted from Bailey SH, Saint-Cyr M, Oni G, et al. The low transverse extended latissimus dorsi flap based on fat compartments of the back for breast reconstruction: anatomical study and clinical results. *Plast Reconstr Surg.* 2011;128:382e-394e, with permission from the American Society of Plastic Surgeons.)

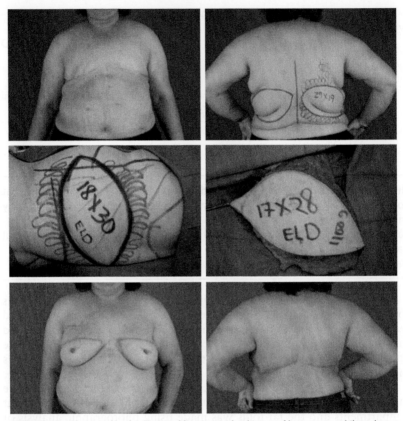

FIGURE 10.—Photographs of a 43-year-old patient with a history of breast cancer, bilateral mastectomies, and radiation therapy. This patient was not a candidate for an abdomen-based flap and underwent surgery for bilateral extended latissimus dorsi flaps, which weighed 1100 g when measured intraoperatively. (Reprinted from Bailey SH, Saint-Cyr M, Oni G, et al. The low transverse extended latissimus dorsi flap based on fat compartments of the back for breast reconstruction: anatomical study and clinical results. *Plast Reconstr Surg.* 2011;128:382e-394e, with permission from the American Society of Plastic Surgeons.)

who had a low transverse extended latissimus dorsi flap performed by the senior author (M.S.-C.).

Results.—Cadaveric dissection and photographic analysis confirmed the presence of the four distinct fat compartments in the back. The lower compartments 3 and 4 were the most frequently identified and the largest, with mean values of 367 cm^3 and 271 cm^3, respectively. The clinical series comprised eight high—body mass index patients who underwent 12 pure autologous breast reconstructions using the low transverse skin paddle harvest technique. Donor-site complications included partial dehiscence ($n = 2$) and minor infection ($n = 3$). There were no instances of seroma, and fat necrosis (<5 percent) occurred in one breast.

Conclusions.—The low transverse skin paddle extended latissimus dorsi flap is reliable and provides sufficient volume for purely autologous breast reconstruction with low donor-site morbidity and improved body contouring for a select group of patients. The authors' initial experience with high—body mass index patients shows promising results with this flap in a challenging group (Figs 1 and 10).

▶ This procedure is a good alternative to the use of abdominal flaps in high-risk patients, the obese, smokers, and others. It is also an option for centers without microsurgical expertise. The authors are to be commended for the identification, anatomical elucidation, and use of the fat compartments adjacent to the latissimus dorsi musculature in the back of obese women for autologous breast reconstruction (Figs 1 and 10). Of course reconstructed breast volume can always be enhanced with the use of fat grafts.

S. H. Miller, MD

Prosthetic Breast Reconstruction After Implant-Sparing Mastectomy in Patients With Submuscular Implants

Suber J, Malafa M, Smith P, et al (Univ of South Florida, Tampa)
Ann Plast Surg 66:546-550, 2011

Women with previous submuscular breast augmentation who contract breast cancer have several options for breast reconstruction. Our institution offers implant-sparing mastectomy with delayed implant exchange. A retrospective review of 10 patients who underwent implant-sparing mastectomies with delayed implant exchange between 2006 and 2010 was performed. The average age at implant exchange was 48.7 years. The average time between initial augmentation and mastectomy was 7.45 years. The average time between mastectomy and implant exchange was 7.1 months. One patient underwent partial mastectomy with radiation. The average size of implant at initial augmentation was 366 mL. The average size of implant exchange on side of mastectomy was 565.5 mL. One patient underwent a second exchange for larger implants. No other complications were noted. Implant-sparing mastectomy with delayed exchange provides an alternative to tissue expander placement and associated morbidities. This technique provides excellent results with minimal complications for this patient population.

▶ Women in whom breast cancer develops after breast augmentation constitute a sometimes challenging group of patients. In most centers, these patients undergo mastectomy (when appropriate) plus implant removal, followed by some form of reconstruction if desired (and most of these patients do desire reconstruction). These authors present an interesting alternative approach in those patients who have undergone augmentation with submuscular implants. The authors advocate a very simple approach: perform the mastectomy while leaving the implant in place, then return later and increase the size of the implant proportional to the amount of breast tissue removed. The results reported and visualized in the article appear to be satisfactory. Some questions are not answered in the article: Were the implants "totally submuscular," so that the capsule around the implant would not be disturbed by a mastectomy? What should be done if the capsule has to be entered? How easy or how difficult was it to place an implant with an average size increase of 200 mL in the existing pocket at a later date? An alternative approach to this problem has been suggested by others—preserve the implant (especially if the capsule has been entered) and augment the existing implant volume with a latissimus dorsi flap (perhaps harvested endoscopically to reduce scar). Both approaches appear to be worthy of consideration, especially if the patient expresses a strong desire to keep her implants.

R. L. Ruberg, MD

The Use of AlloDerm in Postmastectomy Alloplastic Breast Reconstruction: Part I. A Systematic Review
Jansen LA, Macadam SA (Univ of British Columbia, Vancouver, Canada)
Plast Reconstr Surg 127:2232-2244, 2011

Background.—Postmastectomy alloplastic breast reconstruction is a common procedure that continues to evolve. Increasingly, AlloDerm is being used in both direct-to-implant and two-stage breast reconstruction. The objective of this systematic review was to summarize the outcomes from studies describing this use of AlloDerm, and to compare outcomes to those from studies reviewing non-AlloDerm alloplastic reconstruction.

Methods.—A computerized search was performed across multiple databases. Studies involving patients undergoing alloplastic breast reconstruction with AlloDerm were included. A systematic review was performed to include randomized controlled trials, comparative observational studies, noncomparative observational studies, and case series.

Results.—A systematic review of the literature revealed 14 studies that satisfied inclusion criteria. Both acute and long-term complication rates were obtained. No objective validated outcomes were reported. Ninety-three percent of included studies were level IV evidence. Complication rates were as follows: infection, 0 to 11 percent; hematoma, 0 to 6.7 percent; seroma, 0 to 9 percent; partial flap necrosis, 0 to 25 percent; implant exposure with removal, 0 to 14 percent; implant exposure with salvage, 0 to 4 percent; capsular contracture, 0 to 8 percent; and rippling, 0 to 6 percent. No study included a cost analysis.

Conclusions.—Complications using AlloDerm are comparable to those of non-AlloDerm alloplastic reconstructions. AlloDerm appears to confer a low rate of capsular contracture. A formal analysis is required to determine AlloDerm's cost effectiveness in use for direct-to-implant reconstructions. In addition, a randomized controlled trial comparing AlloDerm use to conventional two-stage reconstruction is currently absent from the literature.

▶ I believe that the use of AlloDerm has potential application in breast reconstruction after mastectomy as well as in cosmetic augmentation. However, I must admit, after carefully reading this systematic review, that I would be hard-pressed to document the veracity of my "beliefs." Suffice it to say, "no study used validated or standardized outcome measures." All studies were based on Level IV evidence, and most included few patients. Several studies reported elevation of the serratus muscle, but most did not. Comparisons were historical with 2 other studies, neither of which used AlloDerm. Complication rates and types of complications in each of the studies used to formulate this report could not be adequately assessed or discerned by the authors of this review. If we are to promote the use of this material for breast reconstruction, it is incumbent upon the specialty, or those with the capability to do so, to organize a meaningful prospective and randomized study based on strict protocols for the use of AlloDerm, as well as protocols for data collection of complications and outcomes.

S. H. Miller, MD

A Systematic Review and Meta-Analysis of Complications Associated With Acellular Dermal Matrix-Assisted Breast Reconstruction

Ho G, Nguyen TJ, Shahabi A, et al (Keck School of Medicine of Univ of Southern California, Los Angeles)
Ann Plast Surg 68:346-356, 2012

Background.—Multiple outcome studies have been published on the use of acellular dermal matrix (ADM) in breast reconstruction with disparate results. The purpose of this study was to conduct a systematic review and meta-analysis to determine an aggregate estimate of risks associated with ADM-assisted breast reconstruction.

Methods.—The MEDLINE, Web of Science, and Cochrane Library databases were queried, and relevant articles published up to September 2010 were analyzed based on specific inclusion criteria. Seven complications were studied including seroma, cellulitis, infection, hematoma, skin flap necrosis, capsular contracture, and reconstructive failure. A pooled random effects estimate for each complication and 95% confidence intervals (CI) were derived. For comparisons of ADM and non-ADM, the pooled random effects odds ratio (OR) and 95% CI were derived. Heterogeneity was measured using the I^2 statistic.

Results.—Sixteen studies met the inclusion criteria. The pooled complication rates were seroma (6.9%; 95% CI, 5.3%−8.8%), cellulitis (2.0%; 95% CI, 1.2%−3.1%), infection (5.7%; 95% CI, 4.3%−7.3%), skin flap necrosis (10.9%; 95% CI, 8.7%−13.5%), hematoma (1.3%; 95% CI, 0.6%−2.4%), capsular contracture (0.6%; 95% CI, 0.1%−1.7%), and reconstructive failure (5.1%; 95% CI, 3.8%−6.7%). Five studies reported findings for both the ADM and non-ADM patients and were used in the meta-analysis to calculate pooled OR. ADM-assisted breast reconstructions had a higher likelihood of seroma (pooled OR, 3.9; 95% CI, 2.4−6.2), infection (pooled OR, 2.7; 95% CI, 1.1−6.4), and reconstructive failure (pooled OR, 3.0; 95% CI, 1.3−6.8) than breast reconstructions without the use of ADM. The relation of ADM use to hematoma (pooled OR, 2.0; 95% CI, 0.8−5.2), cellulitis (pooled OR, 2.0; 95% CI, 0.9−4.3), and skin flap necrosis (pooled OR, 1.9; 95% CI, 0.6−5.4) was inconclusive.

Conclusions.—In the studies evaluated, ADM-assisted breast reconstructions exhibited a higher likelihood of seroma, infection, and reconstructive failure than prosthetic-based breast reconstructions using traditional musculofascial flaps. ADM is associated with a lower rate of capsular contracture. A careful risk/benefit analysis should be performed when choosing to use ADM in implant-based breast reconstruction.

▶ It would be worthwhile for all plastic surgeons who perform breast reconstruction to read and carefully study this meta-analysis, along with the earlier study published in *Plastic and Reconstructive Surgery* by Jansen and Macadam.[1] The conclusions in this article are quite different from those of the earlier study in that the risks of seroma, infection, and reconstructive failure were statistically higher. Perhaps this was a result of several factors: differences in both the number and currency of articles included, differences in the acellular dermal matrix product used, and differences in evaluating complication rates. The bottom line is that we are still left with many more questions than answers regarding this product and guidelines for its use. This material must be studied in a prospective and randomized fashion on comparable cohorts of patients undergoing comparable reconstructions (using autologous material vs acellular dermal matrix) and timing (1 stage vs 2 stages). In addition, we must determine if it is safe, what value for the patient is added, and at what cost. Finally, if infection is truly of concern, the producers of the product must develop reliable techniques to ensure its sterility.

S. H. Miller, MD

Reference

1. Jansen LA, Macadam SA. The Use of AlloDerm in postmastectomy alloplastic breast reconstruction: part I A systematic review. *Plast Reconstr Surg.* 2011; 127:2232-2244.

Prospective trial of Adipose-Derived Regenerative Cell (ADRC)-enriched fat grafting for partial mastectomy defects: The RESTORE-2 trial
Pérez-Cano R, Vranckx JJ, Lasso JM, et al (Hospital General Universitario Gregorio Maranon, Madrid, Spain; KU Leuven Univ Hosp, Belgium; et al)
Eur J Surg Oncol 38:382-389, 2012

Aims.—Women undergoing breast conservation therapy (BCT) for breast cancer are often left with contour defects and few acceptable reconstructive options. RESTORE-2 is the first prospective clinical trial using autologous adipose-derived regenerative cell (ADRC)-enriched fat grafting for reconstruction of such defects. This single-arm, prospective, multi-center clinical trial enrolled 71 patients post-BCT with defects ≤150 mL.

Methods.—Adipose tissue was collected via syringe lipoharvest and then processed during the same surgical procedure using a closed automated system that isolates ADRCs and prepares an ADRC-enriched fat graft for immediate re-implantation. ADRC-enriched fat graft injections were performed in a fan-shaped pattern to prevent pooling of the injected fat. Overall procedure times were less than 4 h. The RESTORE-2 protocol allowed for up to two treatment sessions and 24 patients elected to undergo a second procedure following the six month follow-up visit.

Results.—Of the 67 patients treated, 50 reported satisfaction with treatment results through 12 months. Using the same metric, investigators reported satisfaction with 57 out of 67 patients. Independent radiographic core laboratory assessment reported improvement in the breast contour of 54 out of 65 patients based on blinded assessment of MRI sequence. There were no serious adverse events associated with the ADRC-enriched

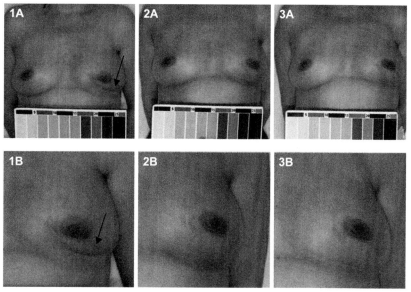

FIGURE 1.—Pre-operative views (1A, 1B) and post-operative views at six (2A, 2B) and 12 months (3A, 3B). This patient presented 28 months following BCT. At time of excision, tumor size measured 0.8 cm in width. Radiation history included 30 treatments with a cumulative dose of 60 Gy. Visual defect estimate at baseline was 100 mL. A total of 385 mL of lipoaspirate was harvested from the abdomen and 150 mL of "wet" ADRC-enriched fat was injected into the left lower pole defect in a single session with a transplantation time of 25 min. At 12 months patient and investigator satisfaction with overall treatment results were reported as "satisfied." (Reprinted from Pérez-Cano R, Vranckx JJ, Lasso JM, et al. Prospective trial of adipose-derived regenerative cell (ADRC)-enriched fat grafting for partial mastectomy defects: the RESTORE-2 trial. *Eur J Surg Oncol.* 2012;38:382-389, Copyright 2012, with permission from Elsevier.)

fat graft injection procedure. There were no reported local cancer recurrences. Injection site cysts were reported as adverse events in ten patients.

Conclusion.—This prospective trial demonstrates the safety and efficacy of the treatment of BCT defects utilizing ADRC-enriched fat grafts (Fig 1).

▶ This is a report of an early prospective European multicenter clinical trial determining the efficacy of using autologous adipose-derived regenerative cells (ADRC) plus lipoaspirate fat for the reconstruction of breast defects following breast conservation and radiotherapy for breast carcinoma. The results reported a high level of satisfaction by patients and an even higher satisfaction level by the investigators. It is unclear whether the investigators both treated and assessed the results (Fig 1). I am also not certain whether the ideal ratio of ADRC tissue to fat aspirate has been determined, but to be fair, perhaps this can be found in another study and just not reported here. As mentioned by the authors, a limitation in the secondary goal of the study was their inability to determine if breast volume, using MRI, changed as a result of the ADRC-enriched fat grafts. Obviously it will be important to determine this and to document whether changes in fact remain stable over time. Finally, it is essential to have a similar study performed in a head-to-head double blind study with non-ADRC-enriched grafts harvested, treated, and injected according to a standardized protocol used by all participants and the results evaluated by patients and noninvestigators as well as reliable measures of changes in breast volume.

S. H. Miller, MD

7 Scars and Wound Healing

Wound Healing

Modern wound care for the poor: a randomized clinical trial comparing the vacuum system with conventional saline-soaked gauze dressings

Perez D, Bramkamp M, Exe C, et al (Hôpital Albert Schweitzer, Deschapelles, Haiti; Univ Hosp of Zurich, Switzerland)

Am J Surg 199:14-20, 2010

Background.—A clinical randomized trial was performed to determine whether a simple homemade wound vacuum-dressing system (HM-VAC) is a feasible alternative to the use of conventional saline-soaked gauze dressings (WET) for the treatment of complex wounds in a resource-poor hospital.

Methods.—Forty patients were analyzed to compare the HM-VAC and the WET dressings. The HM-VAC was assembled with tools available in most operating room worldwide. The primary outcome measure was the time of complete wound healing. Additionally, the costs of both methods were calculated.

Results.—The time required to achieve complete healing was 16 days in the HM-VAC group compared with 25 days in the WET group ($P = .013$). The HM-VAC costs US $360 per case, and the WET technique costs US $271 per case ($P = .008$).

Conclusions.—The HM-VAC should be considered in underdeveloped countries to provide modern management for complex wounds because healing is significantly faster compared with conventional wound care. Although the HM-VAC is more costly than the conventional approach, it is probably affordable for most resource-poor hospitals.

▶ Working in a first-world medical center, we can sometimes forget how lucky we are, for the most part, to have access to the majority of advanced technologies to help our patients. Unfortunately, many areas do not have the same blessings, and they are required to be more imaginative in what they can offer patients. In wound care, vacuum-dressing system (VAC) therapy (KCI Inc, San Antonio) has been revolutionary, but it is expensive, especially in areas with limited resources. This study was an excellent comparative study between a homemade wound vacuum-dressing system (HM-VAC) and standard wet-to-dry dressings. Interestingly, instead of standard scrub sponges, which have been described for other subatmospheric dressings, they used povidone-iodine sponges. There is some controversy as to whether the iodine solution might be slightly toxic to the wound bed, but they showed excellent results compared with standard dressing changes. If one was concerned about the iodine, and no other sponges were available, the surgeon could always irrigate the sponges to dilute the iodine significantly. The authors did a cost analysis, which was inadequate because they could not get cost information from the administration of their hospital (sounds like a problem both first world and third world hospitals have in common), but did show that there was a significantly shortened time of the HM-VAC dressing system to wound closure (16 days vs 25 days) and total hospital stay (83 vs 121 days). Obviously, it would have been good to compare the commercial VAC with the HM-HVAC, but it is reasonable to understand how they did not have access or funds to do that study. It is worthy of applause to see that even in a disadvantaged medical system, academic inquiry and pursuit are attainable.

J. Boehmler, MD

Wound Healing and Infection in Surgery: The Pathophysiological Impact of Smoking, Smoking Cessation, and Nicotine Replacement Therapy: A Systematic Review
Sørensen LT (Univ of Copenhagen, Denmark)
Ann Surg 255:1069-1079, 2012

Objective.—The aim was to clarify how smoking and nicotine affects wound healing processes and to establish if smoking cessation and nicotine replacement therapy reverse the mechanisms involved.

Background.—Smoking is a recognized risk factor for healing complications after surgery, but the pathophysiological mechanisms remain largely unknown.

Methods.—Pathophysiological studies addressing smoking and wound healing were identified through electronic databases (PubMed, EMBASE) and by hand-search of articles' bibliography. Of the 1460 citations identified, 325 articles were retained following title and abstract reviews. In total, 177 articles were included and systematically reviewed.

Results.—Smoking decreases tissue oxygenation and aerobe metabolism temporarily. The inflammatory healing response is attenuated by a reduced inflammatory cell chemotactic responsiveness, migratory function, and oxidative bactericidal mechanisms. In addition, the release of proteolytic enzymes and inhibitors is imbalanced. The proliferative response is impaired by a reduced fibroblast migration and proliferation in addition to a downregulated collagen synthesis and deposition. Smoking cessation restores tissue oxygenation and metabolism rapidly. Inflammatory cell response is reversed in part within 4 weeks, whereas the proliferative response remains impaired.

Nicotine does not affect tissue microenvironment, but appears to impair inflammation and stimulate proliferation.

Conclusions.—Smoking has a transient effect on the tissue microenvironment and a prolonged effect on inflammatory and reparative cell functions leading to delayed healing and complications. Smoking cessation restores the tissue microenvironment rapidly and the inflammatory cellular functions within 4 weeks, but the proliferative response remain impaired. Nicotine and nicotine replacement drugs seem to attenuate inflammation and enhance proliferation but the effect appears to be marginal.

▶ If a plastic surgeon ever wanted to get a good night's sleep, this is the article to cure even the most severe case of insomnia. But despite its narcoleptic properties, it is a fundamentally important review article that plastic surgeons (and all surgeons for that matter) should be familiar with. It gives significant rationale for smoking cessation for at least 4 weeks prior to any significant elective surgery, like facelifts, abdominoplasties, or breast reductions. There are several key points from this review. First, the effect of smoking on perfusion and oxygenation can decrease subcutaneous blood flow by up to 40% but is only limited for a couple of hours. Second, smoking creates significant oxidative stress, which can cause cellular damage and impair cellular function and can last for 2 to 4 weeks. These effects might be partially alleviated with vitamin C and E supplementation, but further study for that is warranted. The effect of smoking that is most likely to be causative of wound healing complications is nicotine's detrimental effect on inflammation and proliferation of the wound healing process. Lastly, there is no consensus about nicotine replacement therapies, like the patch or gum, but it can be considered that the vasoconstrictive properties of nicotine could be detrimental in the peri- and postoperative state. Smoking and nicotine are very harmful to the wound healing capabilities of surgical patients, and smoking cessation for at least 4 weeks will provide the best opportunity for the patient to have a successful and happy outcome.

J. Boehmler, MD

Miscellaneous

The effect of hyperbaric oxygen therapy on the survival of random pattern skin flaps in nicotine-treated rats

Selçuk CT, Kuvat SV, Bozkurt M, et al (Dicle Univ Med Faculty, Diyarbakir, Turkey; Reconstructive and Aesthetic Surgery, Istanbul, Turkey; et al)
J Plast Reconstr Aesthet Surg 65:489-493, 2012

Previous studies have shown that nicotine increases the risk of necrosis in skin flaps. We investigated the effect of hyperbaric oxygen (HBO_2) treatment on the survival of random skin flaps in nicotine-treated rats.

Thirty-two Sprague—Dawley rats were divided into four groups with eight rats in each group. Group 1 ($n = 8$) was the control, group 2 ($n = 8$) received HBO_2 treatment without being exposed to nicotine, group 3 ($n = 8$) received nicotine and group 4 ($n = 8$) received HBO_2 treatment with exposure to nicotine. The rats in the nicotine-treated groups were prepared by treating them with nicotine for 28 days. At the end of the 28th day, standard McFarlane-type random skin flaps were lifted from the backs of all the rats. In groups 2 and 4, HBO_2 treatment started at the 30th min following the surgery and continued once a day for 7 days.

The flap survival rates and histopathological evaluation results related to neovascularisation and granulation tissue formation were significantly better in the HBO_2-treated groups (groups 2 and 4) than in the groups that did not receive HBO_2 treatment (groups 1 and 3) ($p < 0.05$). The flap survival rates, neovascularisation and granulation tissue formation were highest in group 2 and lowest in group 3 ($p \leq 0.001$). No significant difference was observed between group 4, which received HBO_2 treatment with nicotine exposure, and the control group (group 1) ($p > 0.05$).

In conclusion, our study demonstrates that HBO_2 treatment has a positive effect on flap survival in nicotine-treated rats (Fig 1).

▶ Performing random pattern skin flaps on active smokers can certainly be a stressful situation for any plastic surgeon. Despite aggressive counseling and encouragement, many patients will continue to smoke up to and beyond their surgery. Although it may be easier to refuse to do cosmetic surgery on an active smoker, there are situations in which a patient needs to have surgery (eg, cancer, trauma) and plastic surgeons are forced into performing surgery in suboptimal conditions. This article shows very favorable results, albeit in a rat model, for using postoperative hyperbaric oxygen (HBO_2) to improve the survival of random pattern skin flaps. After creating a cohort of nicotine-addicted rats over a 28-day span, they randomized rats to get 7 days of postoperative HBO_2 versus control of no HBO_2 (Fig 1). Although they showed a very significant improvement in flap

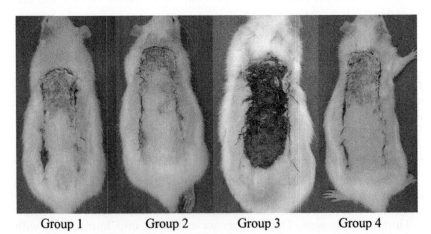

| Group 1 | Group 2 | Group 3 | Group 4 |

FIGURE 1.—Appearance of necrotic and viable skin areas of the flap on postoperative day 7. (Reprinted from Selçuk CT, Kuvat SV, Bozkurt M, et al. The effect of hyperbaric oxygen therapy on the survival of random pattern skin flaps in nicotine-treated rats. *J Plast Reconstr Aesthet Surg*. 2012;65:489-493, Copyright 2012, with permission from British Association of Plastic, Reconstructive and Aesthetic Surgeons.)

survival, there were a couple of shortcomings. First, they administered the initial treatment of HBO_2 within 30 minutes of surgery, which would not be very realistic in a plastic surgery practice. Second, they did not administer any more nicotine after surgery. Surely, although some patients may not smoke after local flap reconstruction, many would, and it would have been interesting to see how administration of HBO_2 and nicotine at the same time postoperatively would have fared. Regardless, if a surgeon encounters a patient who is an active smoker and is not likely to quit before (or after) surgery, making the pre-emptive referral to a HBO_2 unit might make a difference.

J. Boehmler, MD

8 Grafts, Flaps, and Microsurgery

Grafts

Split Skin Graft Application Over an Integrating, Biodegradable Temporizing Polymer Matrix: Immediate and Delayed

Greenwood JE, Dearman BL (Royal Adelaide Hosp, South Australia, Australia)
J Burn Care Res 33:7-19, 2012

The objective of this study is to further investigate the NovoSorb™ biodegradable polyurethane in generating dermal scaffolds; to perform a pilot study comparing the previously used spun mat against a recently developed NovoSorb™ foam, ascertaining the optimum structure of the matrix; and to evaluate the successful matrix as an immediate adjunct to split skin grafting and as a temporizing matrix in a prospective six-pig study. A pilot study comparing a previously investigated form of the polymer (spun mat) against a new structural form, a foam, was performed. This was followed by a six-pig study of the foam matrix with three treatment arms—autologous split skin graft alone, polymer foam with immediate engraftment, and polymer foam with delayed engraftment. The foams allowed less wound contraction than the spun mats. The foam structure is less dense (cheaper to produce and having less degradation products). The material remained in situ despite clinical wound infection. Proof of concept was achieved in both treatment modalities in the main study. Split skin graft applied immediately over the polymer foam was able to engraft successfully. The result was "thicker" to pinch and "flush" with the skin surrounding the wound. There was no significant difference in the degree of wound contraction between the graft alone and the polymer plus immediate graft groups. Split skin graft also "took" when applied to the surface of a polymer that had been applied to a wound 11 days earlier, again with a thicker result, flush with the surrounding skin. Split skin grafts alone left a persisting depression. However, a significant degree of wound contraction (compared with the other two groups) was observed in the polymer plus delayed graft group. This has prompted further investigation into "sealing" the polymer foam with a membrane, to prevent evaporative water loss, when the foam is to be used as a biodegradable temporizing matrix. The studies indicate that the NovoSorb™ platform will allow the creation of two inexpensive dermal matrix products; an immediate scaffold to allow a thicker grafting result and a biodegradable temporizing matrix (BTM) for wound integration after burn debridement while donor sites become reharvestable. However, further modification on the BTM structure is necessary to further reduce wound contraction pregrafting.

▶ In burn care, especially large surface area burns, thin split thickness skin grafts are required to maximally harvest skin from the available donor sites, which can only be harvested a few times. By building a "neo-dermis" to help create thickness in the wound, thinner skin grafts can be harvested while allowing for a more durable final reconstruction, with possibly less wound contraction. Currently, one of the few options for dermal regeneration is use of Integra® biomatrix. Although it is widely used to prepare wound beds for eventual skin grafting, it is unfortunately expensive and prone to infection. This interesting article highlights the potential promises and drawbacks of another methodology, mainly a biodegradable polyurethane polymer. In this porcine study, the matrix (NovoSorb™) was used as a 1-mm dermal-regenerative substrate that was evaluated for its ability to take a skin graft immediately placed on it versus a delayed fashion after allowing for vascular integration. Although their results looked promising in regard to eventual graft take and "skin thickness" in both groups, the wounds had more contraction compared to a control group of skin graft only without the NovoSorb™ matrix. Until this issue of contraction is resolved to be at least equivalent to skin grafting alone, it is hard to appreciate its long-term clinical usefulness. Regardless, this study was a good step forward toward the development of less-expensive, lab-grown substrates that could eventually hold a vital role in the care of burn and wound patients.

J. Boehmler, MD

Recruited Minced Skin Grafting for Improving the Skin Appearance of the Donor Site of a Split-Thickness Skin Graft
Simizu R, Kishi K, Okabe K, et al (Keio Univ, Tokyo, Japan)
Dermatol Surg 38:654-660, 2012

Objective.—To improve skin appearance at the donor site of a split-thickness skin graft, part of the harvested skin was minced and grafted back onto the site in a process we named "recruited minced skin grafting."

Materials and Methods.—Thirteen Japanese patients who needed split-thickness skin grafts were treated with recruited minced skin grafting. Five patients were used as controls, in whom donor sites were treated with the traditional method. Part of the split-thickness skin was minced using two surgical blades (number 24) to an approximate particle size of less than 0.5 mm. Minced skin was spread and transplanted onto the donor site and covered with polyurethane foam. Twelve months after the operation, donor sites were scored for hypopigmentation, hyperpigmentation, redness, and disruption of skin texture. Gross appearance was evaluated according to total score.

Results.—Donor sites treated with recruited minced skin grafts had significantly better appearance than those of controls. Donor sites that had more than 5% of the total area treated tended to have better results.

Conclusion.—Recruited minced skin grafting is a good method of improving the appearance of the donor site (Figs 3 and 4).

▶ This is an interesting concept from a group of Japanese plastic surgeons. Use of minced skin grafts has been reported in a wide variety of situations, including burn wounds, leg ulcers and leukoderma, and depigmentation of the skin. The authors state that in a small group (13 patients) who needed split thickness skin grafts, the cosmetic appearance of the donor site at 12 months, with regard to pigmentation, redness, and skin texture, in those treated with minced skin grafts mixed with prostaglandin and covered with polyurethane foam was better than the donor sites of those who were treated without the minced skin or prostaglandin but merely covered with polyurethane foam. Although the results demonstrated seem to document the authors' conclusions, the results would have been more

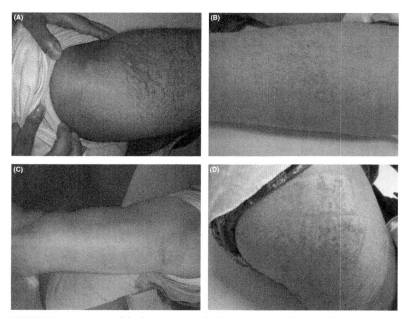

FIGURE 3.—Appearance of the donor site treated with recruited minced skin grafting 12 months after the procedure. (A) Lateral thigh of a 59-year-old man. The contour was nice, and the site had much less hyperpigmentation, hypopigmentation, and redness than typically seen with the traditional method; thus, the donor site was evaluated as excellent. (B) Lateral thigh of a 31-year-old man; the results were evaluated as excellent. (C) Lateral thigh of a 56-year-old man. Partial hypopigmentation (<25%) was observed. The donor site was evaluated as good. (D) Right buttock of a 42-year-old man. Partial hypopigmentation and redness (<25%) were observed. The donor site was evaluated as fair. (Reprinted from Simizu R, Kishi K, Okabe K, et al. Recruited minced skin grafting for improving the skin appearance of the donor site of a split-thickness skin graft. *Dermatol Surg.* 2012;38:654-660, with permission from John Wiley & Sons, Inc.)

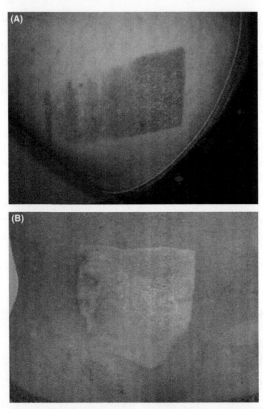

FIGURE 4.—Appearance of the donor site without recruited minced skin grafting 12 months after the procedure. (A) Right lateral thigh of a 51-year-old man. More than 75% of the area became red. The donor site was evaluated as poor. (B) Back of a 41-year-old man. More than 75% of the area became red or hypopigmented. The donor site was evaluated as poor (B). (Reprinted from Simizu R, Kishi K, Okabe K, et al. Recruited minced skin grafting for improving the skin appearance of the donor site of a split-thickness skin graft. *Dermatol Surg*. 2012;38:654-660, with permission from John Wiley & Sons, Inc.)

definitive had the authors been able to divide the wounds on the same person and treated half with the minced grafts and the other half in a standard fashion, especially since the anatomic location of the donor sites and the results achieved varied. Generally, donor sites on the buttocks fared less well than did other sites, even in the minced graft group (Figs 3 and 4).

S. H. Miller, MD

Microsurgery

Development of consensus guidelines for venous thromboembolism prophylaxis in patients undergoing microvascular reconstruction of the mandible

Deleyiannis FW-B, Clavijo-Alvarez JA, Pullikkotil B, et al (Univ of Pittsburgh Med Ctr, PA)
Head Neck 33:1034-1040, 2011

Background.—The purpose of this study was to determine how guidelines for venous thromboembolism prophylaxis can be applied to patients undergoing microsurgical reconstruction of the mandible.

Methods.—Retrospective review of our institutional use of thromboprophylaxis and the associated outcomes in 114 patients (58 free fibular flaps and 56 osteocutaneous radial forearm flaps).

Results.—Twenty-two patients (19.3%) received only intermittent pneumatic compression. Overall, 80.7% received postoperative chemoprophylaxis. Sixty-four percent initiated chemoprophylaxis within 24 hours after surgery. Only 13.2% received the recommended frequency of chemoprophylaxis. One patient had development of a pulmonary embolism. Four patients undergoing chemoprophylaxis had development of neck hematomas; in each case the cause of bleeding could be attributed to a cause distinct from chemoprophylaxis.

Conclusions.—No consistent chemoprophylaxis protocol was followed. Chemoprophylaxis was not associated with an increased risk of bleeding. Physician education is the next step in decreasing variations in chemoprophylaxis and adopting guidelines similar to The American College of Chest Physicians.

▶ This is the first study that has critically examined the adherence to American College of Chest Physicians (ACCP) guidelines for patients undergoing osteocutaneous free flap reconstruction. No consistent chemoprophylaxis protocol was followed. Only a minority of the patients received the recommended frequency or time of initiation of therapy of chemoprophylaxis that would have been recommended for a patient undergoing high-risk general orthopedic surgery. The authors advocate the adoption of the ACCP guidelines until further specific information is available for free flap surgery. We must all evaluate our adherence to these guidelines. These will become increasingly important.

D. J. Smith, Jr, MD

Medicinal leeches and the microsurgeon: a four-year study, clinical series and risk benefit review
Whitaker IS, Josty IC, Hawkins S, et al (Morriston Hosp, Swansea, UK; et al)
Microsurgery 31:281-287, 2011

Background.—There are case reports and small series in the literature relating to the use of medicinal leeches by plastic surgeons; however, larger series from individual units are rare. The aim of this article is to present a comprehensive 4-year case series of the use of medicinal leeches, discuss the current evidence regarding indications, risks, and benefits and highlight the recent updates regarding leech speciation.

Methods.—Patients prescribed leeches in a 4-year period (July 2004–2008) were collated from hospital pharmacy records ($N = 35$). The number of leeches used, demographic, clinical, and microbiological details were retrospectively analyzed.

Results.—Thirty-five patients were treated with leeches. The age range was 2 to 98 years (mean $= 49.3$). Leeches were most commonly used for venous congestion in pedicled flaps and replantations. Blood transfusions were necessary in 12 cases (34%) [mean $= 2.8$ units, range 2–5 units]. Our infection rate was 20% (7/35) including five infections with Aeromonas spp. (14.2%). The proportion of patients becoming infected after leech therapy was significantly greater in the group of patients that did not receive prophylactic antibiotic treatment (Fisher's Exact test $P = 0.0005$). In total, 14 cases (40%) were salvaged in entirety, in 7 cases 80% or more, in 2 cases 50 to 79%, and in 1 case less than 50% of the tissues were salvaged. In 11 cases (31%), the tissues were totally lost.

Conclusion.—Our study highlights both the benefits and the risks to patients in selected clinical situations and also the potential risks. The routine use of antibiotic prophylaxis is supported. In view of the emerging evidence that *Hirudo verbana* are now used as standard leech therapy, and the primary pathogen is *Aeromonas veronii*, until a large prospective multicenter study is published, large series of patients treated with leeches should be reported.

▶ Medicinal leech therapy is a generally accepted treatment for venous congestion. These authors thoroughly review their series of patients who required leeches. The strength of the article is the thoroughness of the review. It is a must read for anyone who uses or contemplates using leeches. Also, look for their follow-up as they study these patients prospectively.

D. J. Smith, Jr, MD

Technology-assisted and sutureless microvascular anastomoses: evidence for current techniques

Pratt GF, Rozen WM, Westwood A, et al (Univ of Melbourne, Victoria, Australia)
Microsurgery 32:68-76, 2012

Background.—Since the birth of reconstructive microvascular surgery, attempts have been made to shorten the operative time while maintaining patency and efficacy. Several devices have been developed to aid microsurgical anastomoses. This article investigates each of the currently available technologies and attempts to provide objective evidence supporting their use.

Methods.—Techniques of microvascular anastomosis were investigated by performing searches of the online databases Medline and Pubmed. Returned results were assessed according to the criteria for ranking medical evidence advocated by the Oxford Centre for Evidence Based Medicine. Emphasis was placed on publications with quantifiable endpoints such as unplanned return to theatre, flap salvage, and complication rates.

Results.—There is a relative paucity of high-level evidence supporting any form of assisted microvascular anastomosis. Specifically, there are no randomized prospective trials comparing outcomes using one method versus any other. However, comparative retrospective cohort studies do exist and have demonstrated convincing advantages of certain techniques. In particular, the Unilink™/3M™ coupler and the Autosuture™ Vessel Closure System® (VCS®) clip applicator have been shown to have level 2b evidence supporting their use, meaning that the body of evidence achieves a level of comparative cohort studies.

Conclusion.—Of the available forms of assisted microvascular anastomoses, there is level 2b evidence suggesting a positive outcome with the use of the Unilink™/3™ coupler and the Autosuture™ VCS® clip applicator. Other techniques such as cyanoacrylates, fibrin glues, the Medtronic™ U-ClipA®, and laser bonding have low levels of evidence supporting their use. Further research is required to establish any role for these techniques.

▶ This article investigates several devices used to aid microsurgical anastomoses. Of the available forms of assisted microvascular anastomoses, there is level 2b evidence suggesting a positive outcome with the use of the Unilink™/3M™ coupler and the Autosuture™ VCS® clip applicator. Other techniques such as cyanoacrylates, fibrin glues, the Medtronic™ U-Clip®, and laser bonding have low levels of evidence supporting their use. With the increased focus on devices to shorten operating time while maintaining patency, (*see accompanying abstract), it is important to keep focus on the validity of the evidence. Too frequently, large series, poorly controlled, skew the researcher's impression. This is an excellent review both of the devices and the level of evidence.

*Also read: Microvascular anastomosis using the vascular closure device in free flap reconstructive surgery: A 13-year experience.[1]

D. J. Smith, Jr, MD

Reference

1. Reddy C, Pennington D, Stern H. Microvascular anastomosis using the vascular closure device in free flap reconstructive surgery: A 13-year experience. *J Plast Reconstr Aesthet Surg.* 2012;65:195-200.

Microvascular anastomosis using the vascular closure device in free flap reconstructive surgery: A 13-year experience
Reddy C, Pennington D, Stern H (Royal Prince Alfred Hosp, Sydney, Australia)
J Plast Reconstr Aesthet Surg 65:195-200, 2012

The achievement of patency of the microvascular anastomosis in free flap surgery is dependent on a number of factors, central to which is atraumatic handling of the vessel lumen, and intimal apposition. Initial laboratory studies demonstrating the superiority of the non-penetrating vascular closure staple (VCS − Anastoclip®) were followed by our report in 1999 on a series of free flaps. There is still a paucity of data in the literature on the use of non-penetrating devices for microvascular anastomosis, and our review gives evidence to support the routine use of the VCS in microsurgical free flap surgery. We now report on its successful use over a thirteen year period in 819 free flap reconstructions. Our data indicates the VCS device to be as effective as sutured anastomoses in free tissue transfer surgery. There is also statistically significant data (Barnard's Exact Test) to demonstrate a higher vascular patency rate of the VCS device over sutured anastomoses when sub group analysis is performed. 'Take-back' revision rates were lower amongst flaps that employed VCS use. For arterial anastomoses, this equated to 3/654 (0.05%) vs 4/170 (2.4%) with hand-sewn anastomoses ($p = 0.02$). Similarly, for venous anastomoses the 'take-back' revision rate was 7/661 (1.1%) vs 8/165 (4.8%) with hand-sewn anastomoses ($p = 0.003$). Furthermore, the major advantage of the VCS is reduction in anastomosis time, from approximately 25 min per anastomosis for sutures to between five and 10 min for staples.

▶ This is a follow-up report to a 1999 series of free flaps done with a nonpenetrating vascular closure staple. The size of the series, 819 free flaps over a 13-year period, is impressive. Unfortunately, there was no randomization or stratification to understand when the device was, or should be, used. This article suffers from the lack of evidence-based analysis referenced in the previous abstract.

Also read the article: Technology-assisted and sutureless microvascular anastomoses: Evidence for current techniques.[1]

D. J. Smith, Jr, MD

Reference

1. Pratt GF, Rozen WM, Westwood A, et al. Technology-assisted and sutureless microvascular anastomoses: evidence for current techniques. *Microsurgery.* 2012;32:68-76.

The Effect of Neoadjuvant versus Adjuvant Irradiation on Microvascular Free Flap Reconstruction in Sarcoma Patients

Chao AH, Chang DW, Shuaib SW, et al (The Univ of Texas MD Anderson Cancer Ctr, Houston)
Plast Reconstr Surg 129:675-682, 2012

Background.—Sarcoma patients often require radiation therapy in addition to surgical resection. Although neoadjuvant irradiation possesses advantages over adjuvant irradiation related to smaller doses and field sizes, existing studies suggest adverse effects on wound healing and possibly microvascular free flap success. Conversely, microvascular reconstruction may counteract some of the negative effects of irradiation by replacing irradiated tissue with well-vascularized unirradiated tissue from a distant site.

Methods.—A review of sarcoma patients who underwent resection, microsurgical reconstruction, and either neoadjuvant or adjuvant irradiation was performed.

Results.—A total of 119 patients met inclusion criteria, of which 73 underwent neoadjuvant irradiation and 46 underwent adjuvant irradiation. Sarcomas were located in the head and neck ($n = 47$), trunk ($n = 7$), upper extremity ($n = 15$), and lower extremity ($n = 50$). The rate of perioperative (≤ 30 days) complications was 26.9 percent, whereas the rate of late recipient-site complications was 14.3 percent. No significant differences in perioperative recipient-site ($p = 0.19$), donor-site ($p = 1.00$), or medical complications ($p = 0.30$) were observed between patients undergoing neoadjuvant and adjuvant irradiation. Free flap loss rates were lower in patients undergoing neoadjuvant irradiation (0 percent versus 8.7 percent, respectively; $p = 0.02$). Late recipient-site complications occurred less often in patients undergoing neoadjuvant radiation (6.8 percent versus 26.1 percent, respectively; $p = 0.006$).

Conclusions.—Neoadjuvant irradiation does not increase the risk of acute wound or microvascular complications when combined with free flap reconstruction, and is associated with fewer late recipient-site complications than adjuvant irradiation. These factors should be considered when determining the timing of radiation therapy in sarcoma patients undergoing oncologic resections and microsurgical reconstruction.

Clinical Question/Level of Evidence.—Therapeutic, III.

▶ In the treatment of sarcomas, radiation therapy is a frequently utilized treatment modality. Timing of radiation to preoperative (neoadjuvant) versus postoperative (adjuvant) therapy is an area of great debate within the oncologic community. Historically, plastic surgeons may have been reticent about operating in areas that have been previously radiated, especially in microsurgery cases in which the recipient vessels have been radiated. This study is one step in the right direction to dispel these concerns. Neoadjuvant radiation therapy has the distinct advantage of requiring a lesser total radiation dose in a smaller field compared with adjuvant radiation. The benefit of this is potentially decreasing long-term sequela. Although it is difficult to get adequate numbers to give the study appropriate statistical power (given the low numbers of sarcoma patients annually), there is a definite benefit of neoadjuvant radiation therapy for sarcoma patients, especially in the lower extremity, in which they showed a decreased rate of total complications (12.8% for neoadjuvant radiation therapy vs 45.4% for adjuvant). They also displayed a decreased rate of lymphedema with neoadjuvant radiation. In addition, there was no difference in partial or total flap loss in either group, showing that with modern microsurgical techniques, flap reconstruction can be performed safely in the radiated patient.

J. Boehmler, MD

Intravenous Fluid Infusion Rate in Microsurgical Breast Reconstruction: Important Lessons Learned From 354 Free Flaps

Zhong T, Neinstein R, Massey C, et al (Univ Health Network, Toronto, Ontario, Canada; Univ of Toronto, Ontario, Canada; Univ of California at Los Angeles; et al)
Plast Reconstr Surg 128:1153-1160, 2011

Background.—The purpose of this study was to determine the role of intravenous fluid infusion rate in the development of in-hospital complications in patients undergoing microsurgical breast reconstruction for breast cancer.

Methods.—A retrospective review was performed between 2002 and 2009 at a single institution for all consecutive patients undergoing free flap reconstruction of the breast. The authors examined patient variables (age; body mass index; preoperative hemoglobin, hematocrit, and creatinine levels; American Society of Anesthesiologists classification; and cardiac risk factors), surgical variables (type of reconstruction, timing, laterality, need for blood transfusion, and duration of general anesthesia), and fluid variables (rate of crystalloid and colloid infusion in the first 24 hours standardized by weight). The primary outcome was in-hospital complications. The impact of each factor was first determined using univariate tests. The final multivariate logistic regression model was compiled based on variables found to be significant from the univariate analysis and variables felt a priori to affect complication rates.

Results.—Of the 260 patients who had a total of 354 free flaps for breast reconstruction, 54 (20.8 percent) had postoperative complications. There were 40 surgical complications (15.4 percent) and 11 medical complications (4.2 percent), and three patients (1.2 percent) had both types. Most complications were flap related (7.3 percent), including two total flap losses (0.8 percent). Multivariate analysis suggested that the extremes of crystalloid infusion rate significantly predicted postoperative complications ($p = 0.03$) after adjusting for the effect of other covariates.

Conclusion.—This is the first study to report that crystalloid infusion rate, a modifiable variable, is an important predictor of postoperative complications following microsurgical breast reconstruction.

Clinical Question/Level of Evidence.—Risk, III.

▶ Understanding the variables that affect outcome in free flap surgery for breast reconstruction is essential to any surgeon performing these operations. The authors evaluate fluid management, a relatively underexplored area in microsurgery. Multivariate analysis suggested that the extremes of crystallized infusion rate significantly predicted postoperative complications. Fluid overload also has no beneficial effects. Anyone doing free flap breast reconstruction should review this article. While the shortcomings in the methodology are nicely outlined, the basic tenet is sound. This provides appropriate information for a constructive conversation with your anesthetists.

D. J. Smith, Jr, MD

A Cadaver Study of the Vascular Territories of Dominant and Nondominant Internal Mammary Artery Perforators

Paes EC, Schellekens PPA, Hage JJ, et al (Univ Med Ctr Utrecht, The Netherlands; Netherlands Cancer Inst-Antoni van Leeuwenhoek Hosp, Amsterdam, The Netherlands; et al)
Ann Plast Surg 67:68-72, 2011

The perfusion territory of the pedicled internal mammary artery perforator flap has been described, but the number of perforators to be included in the flap's pedicle is controversial. We studied the vascular territory of the dominant perforator and the contribution of additional nondominant perforators to it. Therefore, the dominant perforators in 9 fresh cadavers and the nondominant perforators in 4 of these, were injected with water-based ink. The dominant perforator vascularized a territory extending from the superior border of the clavicle to the xiphoid, and from midsternal to the anterior axial fold, with a mean craniocaudal length of 19.4 cm (range, 17.0–24.0) and a mean mediolateral width of 18.6 cm (range, 16.0–22.5). Additional injection of nondominant perforators did not lead to any substantial enlargement of this territory. One single dominant perforator vascularizes a large part of the hemithorax, allowing for various flap designs. Nondominant perforators do not have to be included in the vascular pedicle of the internal mammary artery perforator flap, which leads to less donor-site morbidity (Fig 1).

▶ This cadaveric injection study is confirmatory of the utility of the internal mammary artery perforator (IMAP) flap. Even though this flap is a variation on the well-known deltopectoral flap, having the anatomic confidence to dissect it onto its dominant vascular pedicle can greatly improve the aesthetic result of the flap and donor site. In this group of 18 flaps, the second intercostal perforator was the dominant perforator in 83% of the specimens and could be identified by CT angiogram or duplex ultrasonography. There was a high surface area of flap perfusion based on the dominant perforator between 300 and 400 cm^2 (Fig 4 in

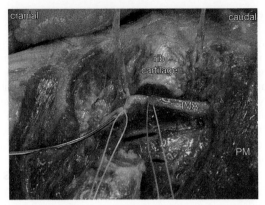

FIGURE 1.—The internal mammary artery (IMA) was approached by dissection of the pectoralis major (PM) and intercostal muscles and the adjacent rib cartilage. The IMA was cannulated and tied off both cranially and caudally to the dominant perforator to prevent leakage and diffusion of the ink through the other perforators. (Reprinted from Paes EC, Schellekens PPA, Hage JJ, et al. A cadaver study of the vascular territories of dominant and nondominant internal mammary artery perforators. *Ann Plast Surg.* 2011;67:68-72, with permission from Lippincott Williams & Wilkins.)

the original article), which generally covered the area between the clavicle to xiphoid and midline to anterior axillary line. Because of this, the flap could be considered a good option as a pedicled or free flap when a large amount of skin is needed, although the donor site would require grafting unless preoperative expansion is considered.

J. Boehmler, MD

Inferior alveolar nerve reconstruction with interpositional sural nerve graft: A sensible addition to one-stage mandibular reconstruction

Chang Y-M, Rodriguez ED, Chu Y-M, et al (Chang Gung Univ Med College, Taipei, Taiwan)
J Plast Reconstr Aesthet Surg 65:757-762, 2012

Background.—This study was to evaluate the sensory recovery in the lower lip and chin in patients who underwent segmental mandibulectomy involving inferior alveolar nerve and simultaneous reconstruction with fibular osteoseptocutaneous flap and interposition sural nerve graft.

Material and Method.—From 1993 to 2004, a total of 20 patients underwent segmental mandibulectomy, simultaneous fibula osteoseptocutaneous flap reconstruction and interpositional sural nerve graft. Twelve patients were available for the study. There were seven male and five female patients with average age of 35.8 years (16−52 years). The sense at the lower lip and chin was measured by two-point discrimination both at the operated and non-operated side at an average of 64.3 months (12−146 months).

Result.—The operated side revealed an average of 13.7 mm for static (STPD) and 13.3 mm for moving two-point discrimination (MTPD) at the lower lip and 13.7 mm for static and 13.4 mm for MTPD at the chin. Data from the non-operated side averaged 3.4 mm for static and 3.2 mm for MTPD at lower lip and 5.1 mm for static and 4.5 mm for moving discrimination at the chin. All patients recovered better than protective sensation on the operated side, which was sufficient to prevent self-mutilation, preserve comprehensible speech and maintain oral competence. No patient complained of significant donor site morbidity.

Conclusion.—Simultaneous reconstruction of a segmental mandibulectomy involving inferior alveolar nerve with a fibula osteoseptocutaneous flap and interpositional sural nerve graft offers simultaneous replacement of mandibular architecture and restoration of protective perioral sensation.

▶ The authors evaluate the sensory recovery in the lower lip and chin in patients who underwent segmental mandibulectomy involving inferior alveolar nerve and simultaneous reconstruction with fibular osteoseptocutaneous flap and interposition sural nerve graft. They conclude that this method is effective in reconstructing patients with benign disease. Patients diagnosed with malignant disease (especially those undergoing radiation) are not suited for this procedure. Patients recovered better than protective sensation in the operated side, which was sufficient to prevent self-mutilation, preserve comprehensible speech, and maintain oral competence. This is a nice modification for anyone doing head and neck reconstruction.

D. J. Smith, Jr, MD

Descending Geniculate Artery: The Ideal Recipient Vessel for Free Tissue Transfer Coverage of Below-the-Knee Amputation Wounds
Higgins JP (Union Memorial Hosp, Baltimore, MD)
J Reconstr Microsurg 27:525-530, 2011

The descending geniculate artery has received notoriety as the source vessel of the medial femoral condyle vascularized bone flap in recent years. Its size and location enable it to serve as a useful recipient vessel in free flap reconstruction about the knee. It is particularly useful in coverage of unstable below-the-knee amputation stumps when recipient vessels are limited. It provides the ease and convenience of two-team surgery in the supine position and its distal position permits convenient and distal insetting of the transferred flap of choice. A discussion of its use in this setting and exemplary cases are provided.

▶ Coverage of distal below-the-knee (BKA) stump wounds with free flaps can be troublesome when considering recipient vessels. This article describes the use of the descending genicular vascular pedicle as a recipient vessel for microsurgical anastomosis. These vessels have been recently popularized because of increased interest in the medial epicondyle cortical periosteal flap. Although this article describes several successful anterolateral thigh (ALT) flap reconstructions with end-to-end anastomoses, it is never discussed what the average diameter of these vessels are. Regardless, as part of an algorithm looking for recipient vessels, the same exposure for the descending genicular vessels could be extended and used for the superficial femoral vessels if the former are not of adequate caliber. Also, these recipient vessels should be considered for cases of proximal leg coverage where there might be only single-vessel runoff to the remainder of the lower extremity, thereby preventing an end-to-side anastomosis to the remaining vessel to the foot, and subsequent potential morbidity if a thrombotic event should occur.

J. Boehmler, MD

Arginine Improves Microcirculation in the Free Transverse Rectus Abdominis Myocutaneous Flap after Breast Reconstruction: A Randomized, Double-Blind Clinical Trial
Booi DI, Debats IBJG, Deutz NEP, et al (Maastricht Univ Med Ctr, The Netherlands)
Plast Reconstr Surg 127:2216-2223, 2011

Background.—Partial flap loss is caused by the incapability of the vascular pedicle to provide sufficient microvascular perfusion in distal segments of the flap in addition to the reperfusion injury that occurs in the whole flap after free tissue transfer. In experimental studies, the amino acid arginine reduces reperfusion injury and improves microvascular perfusion. The purpose of this clinical study was to explore the effect of arginine in free flap surgery.

Methods.—In this randomized, double blind, placebo-controlled trial, 20 patients with unilateral breast reconstruction using the free transverse rectus abdominis myocutaneous flap were included. Patient and flap data were recorded. Patients received a continuous intravenous infusion of arginine or the control amino acid alanine for 5 days. Microcirculation was recorded in the flap in a standardized fashion using laser Doppler flowmetry (Perimed).

Results.—Zone IV microcirculatory blood flow postoperatively was higher in the arginine group than in the alanine control group ($p = 0.04$).

Conclusion.—The authors' study shows beneficial effects of intravenous therapy with arginine to improve microcirculation in the free transverse rectus abdominis myocutaneous flap.

▶ An interesting small double-blinded study, attempting to document that the amino acid arginine, in animal studies, would improve the microcirculation of free transverse rectus abdominis flaps in humans. The authors chose to administer arginine continuously intravenously over 5 days and alanine, for the control solution, in a like manner. Solutions were prepared by a pharmacist, and their contents were unknown to the operating surgeons. Doppler blood flow was higher in Zone IV in the arginine-treated group and major flap loss was more frequent in the alanine (control)-treated group. However, 2 of the 10 flaps in the patients treated with arginine failed, due to anastomosis failure. There were several differences in the 2 study groups, albeit not statistically different because of small numbers in each group; flaps in the alanine group tended to weigh almost 200 grams more than in the arginine group, and the incidence of radiation and chemotherapy was much higher in the alanine group. One wonders whether the results would have been better if the authors had considered using the deep inferior epigastric artery perforator flap or at least not including Zone IV of the transverse rectus abdominis myocutaneous flap. Additionally, might higher doses of arginine and/or the addition of antioxidants or flap delay reduce the incidence of partial flap loss and fat necrosis in these flaps?

S. H. Miller, MD

9 Miscellaneous

Telemedicine and plastic surgery: A review of its applications, limitations and legal pitfalls
Gardiner S, Hartzell TL (Addenbrooke's Hosp, Cambridge, UK; Massachusetts General Hosp, Boston)
J Plast Reconstr Aesthet Surg 65:e47-e53, 2012

Background.—Telemedicine is a rapidly expanding technology involving the exchange of medical information to assist diagnosis and treatment at a distance. Within the field of plastic surgery, where visual examination contributes heavily to patient management decision-making, telemedicine has great potential. However, privacy and medico-legal issues must be considered when using electronic communication to assist our clinical practice.

Methods.—A comprehensive literature review of manuscripts published on telemedicine was performed. Articles were selected for relevance to plastic and reconstructive surgery and reviewed for applications, benefits and complications of telemedicine. In addition, the manuscripts were reviewed for conforming to current legal guidelines for the electronic transfer of patient information.

Results.—Twenty-nine articles met the inclusion criteria (11 trauma and burns, 4 hand, 5 wound-care, 5 maxillofacial, 1 digital replantation, 2 free-flap monitoring, and 1 technical application). Twenty-eight (96%) manuscripts reported a benefit of telemedicine (commonly including increased access to expertise and costs saved through reduction of unnecessary transfers). However only five (17%) reported a statistical benefit compared to a standard treatment cohort (face-to-face interactions). Fifteen (51%) reported on adverse effects, which included misdiagnosis, time consumption, training, technical and cost issues. Only four manuscripts (14%) discussed conforming to legal guidelines within their institution.

Conclusions.—Telemedicine can improve access to the specialty of plastic surgery by facilitating the provision of expertise at remote sites. Its application can be used in many situations and between a variety of healthcare professionals. However, there is little critical analysis on the benefits and risks of telemedicine. In addition, its legal implications need to be carefully considered if it is to be safely integrated into our daily practice.

▶ Use of electronic and digital communications is becoming more accepted, and in some areas is expected between patients and physicians as well as between physicians and other health care providers. Used properly, there can be improved communication and efficiency for all parties involved. Telemedicine is easier with established and noncomplicated patients than with new or complicated cases but can be applied in a large range of clinical problems. Before incorporating these different technologies into practice, institutional, state, and federal regulations must be reviewed (which may not have caught up with current applications). The American Society of Plastic Surgeons offers guiding principles for online communications with patients.[1]

K. A. Gutowski, MD

Reference

1. American Society of Plastic Surgeons. ASPS Guiding Principles: Online Communication for Plastic Surgeons. September 2010. http://www.plasticsurgery.org/Documents/medical-professionals/health-policy/guiding-principles/Online_Communication_for_Plastic_Surgeons_Guiding_Principles.pdf.

An Update on Facial Transplantation Cases Performed between 2005 and 2010
Siemionow M, Ozturk C (Cleveland Clinic, OH)
Plast Reconstr Surg 128:707e-720e, 2011

Background.—Since 2005, 13 facial allotransplantation cases have been performed worldwide. The major indications for these facial allotransplantations were neurofibromatosis and trauma injuries, including animal bites, burns, falls, and shotgun blasts.

Methods.—An analysis of 13 facial transplantation cases was performed by reviewing the anatomical details, microsurgical techniques, and functional outcomes according to the follow-up information based on the literature, meeting presentations, and media reports.

Results.—The male-to-female ratio was 11:2. Two male patients died at 2 months and 2 years, respectively, after transplantation because of transplant- and infection-related problems. Eleven face transplant recipients are alive. The composite tissue allotransplants included cutaneous, myocutaneous, and osteomyocutaneous components. Most of these facial allotransplants were partial, one was nearly total, and two were announced as total face transplantations.

Conclusions.—This report provides a useful overview of the technical aspects of face transplantation; however, the reports on long-term functional and aesthetic outcomes will help to define the future of face transplantation.

▶ This is a very exciting and game-changing technical advance in health care. Of concern is the 15% mortality rate. However, even more disconcerting is that the current state of data gathering and best practices is in an infantile state and frankly of little use to new medical centers and investigators looking to participate in this type of surgery. It is critical, in my opinion, that a worldwide effort be made to develop, agree upon, and use a standardized protocol to record technical data such as tissues transplanted, vascular anastomosis and techniques used, sensory and motor neurological recovery recorded for each procedure, and, perhaps most importantly, appropriate immunologic after care. It is only through such an effort that best practices will emerge.

S. H. Miller, MD

Three Patients with Full Facial Transplantation
Pomahac B, Pribaz J, Eriksson E, et al (Brigham and Women's Hosp, Boston, MA; et al)
N Engl J Med 366:715-722, 2012

Unlike conventional reconstruction, facial transplantation seeks to correct severe deformities in a single operation. We report on three patients who received full-face transplants at our institution in 2011 in operations that aimed for functional restoration by coaptation of all main available motor and sensory nerves. We enumerate the technical challenges and postoperative complications and their management, including single episodes of acute rejection in two patients. At 6 months of followup, all facial allografts were surviving, facial appearance and function were improved, and glucocorticoids were successfully withdrawn in all patients (Fig 1).

▶ This article is a worthwhile read for anyone interested in the world of facial transplantation. The authors have managed to condense a great deal of information into a relatively short article, and the results achieved are quite impressive (Fig 1). The need to tailor the recovery of donor tissues to maximize the benefits for the recipient are discussed, but of course in less detail than one might like. The availability of a supplemental appendix and the video at the *New England Journal of Medicine*'s website are valuable accompaniments to the actual article. Many questions remain to be answered regarding the efficacy, safety, and availability of partial and full face transplants. One can only hope that those involved in advancing these techniques will keep us all regularly informed about the outcomes.

S. H. Miller, MD

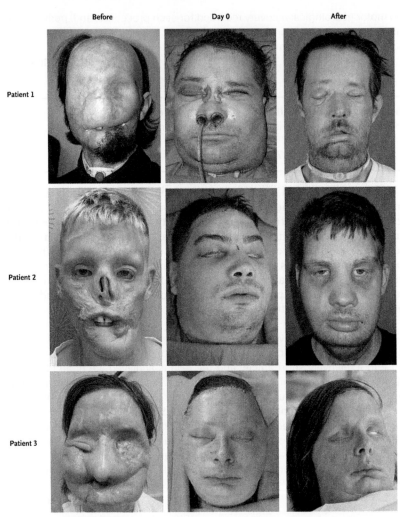

FIGURE 1.—Photographs of the Three Patients before Transplantation and Immediately and Several Months after Surgery. Shown is the preoperative appearance (left column), immediate postoperative appearance (middle column), and appearance after surgery (right column) at 4 months (Patient 1), 3 months (Patient 2), and 2 months (Patient 3). All patients provided written consent for publication of their photographs. (Reprinted from Pomahac B, Pribaz J, Eriksson E, et al. Three patients with full facial transplantation. *N Engl J Med*. 2012;366:715-722, with permission from Massachusetts Medical Society.)

Article Index

Chapter 1: Congenital

Chapter 2: Neoplastic, Inflammatory and Degenerative Conditions

Chapter 3: Trauma

Chapter 4: Hand and Upper Extremity

Chapter 5: Aesthetic

Chapter 6: Breast

Chapter 7: Scars and Wound Healing

Chapter 8: Grafts, Flaps, and Microsurgery

Chapter 9: Miscellaneous

Author Index

Printed and bound by CPI Group (UK) Ltd, Croydon, CR0 4YY

08/05/2025

01864755-0001